OVERVIEW-MAP KEY

OTHER MENASHA RIDGE PRESS PADDLING GUIDES

The Alaska River Guide
Canoeing & Kayaking Florida
Canoeing & Kayaking Georgia
A Canoeing & Kayaking Guide to the Ozarks
A Canoeing & Kayaking Guide to the Streams of Kentucky
Canoeing & Kayaking New York
Canoeing & Kayaking West Virginia
Carolina Whitewater
Paddling the Everglades Wilderness Waterway

PADDLING
LONG ISLAND
AND NEW YORK CITY

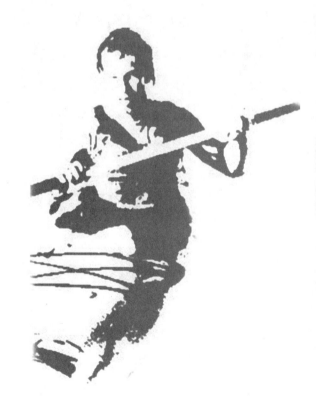

For AnnaGrace and William, with all my love.

—K.S.

PADDLING
LONG ISLAND
AND NEW YORK CITY

The Best Sea Kayaking From
MONTAUK *to* MANHASSET BAY
to MANHATTAN

Kevin Stiegelmaier

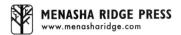 MENASHA RIDGE PRESS
www.menasharidge.com

PADDLING LONG ISLAND AND NEW YORK CITY

Copyright © 2012 by Kevin Stiegelmaier
All rights reserved
Printed in the United States of America
Published by Menasha Ridge Press
Distributed by Publishers Group West
First edition, first printing

Library of Congress Cataloging-in-Publication Data

Stiegelmaier, Kevin.
  Paddling Long Island and New York City : the best sea kayaking from Montauk to
  Manhasset Bay to Manhattan / Kevin Stiegelmaier.
    p. cm.
  ISBN-13: 978-0-89732-529-5 (pbk.)
  ISBN-10: 0-89732-529-X ()
  1. Sea kayaking—New York (State)—Long Island—Guidebooks. 2. Canoes and
  canoeing—New York (State—Long Island—Guidebooks. 3. Sea kayaking—New York
  (State)—New York—Guidebooks. 4. Canoes and canoeing—New York (State)—
  Long Island—Guidebooks. 5. Long Island (N.Y.)—Guidebooks. 6. New York (N.Y.)—
  Guidebooks. I. Title.
  GV776.N7S76 2012
  797.122'40974721—dc23
                                            2012005667

Editors: Ritchey Halphen and Susan Haynes
Cover design: Scott McGrew
Maps: Scott McGrew and Kevin Stiegelmaier
Text design: Alian Design
Cover and interior photos: Kevin Stiegelmaier
Author photo: Laura Stiegelmaier
Photo editor–proofreader: Donna Poehner
Indexer: Ann Cassar/Cassar Technical Services

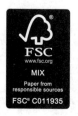
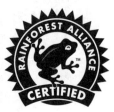

Menasha Ridge Press
P.O. Box 43673
Birmingham, AL 35243
menasharidge.com

DISCLAIMER

This book is meant only as a guide to select paddles on Long Island and does not guarantee your safety in any way—you paddle at your own risk. Neither Menasha Ridge Press nor Kevin Stiegelmaier is liable in any way for property loss or damage, personal injury, or death that may result from accessing or paddling the waterways described in the following pages. Please read carefully the introduction to this book as well as safety information from other sources. Familiarize yourself with current weather reports, maps of the areas you intend to visit (in addition to the maps in this guidebook), and any relevant park regulations. While every effort has been made to ensure the accuracy of this guidebook, water, land, and road conditions, phone numbers and websites, and other information can change from year to year.

CONTENTS

ACKNOWLEDGMENTS

Writing a paddling guidebook is a monumental task that simply cannot be accomplished without the help of others. To the many people who lent me a hand throughout the process, providing assistance, company, or advice whenever it was needed, I owe you all a huge debt of gratitude.

First, I'd like to thank Molly Merkle for giving me the opportunity to write this book and Bob Sehlinger, Ritchey Halphen, and the other editors at Menasha Ridge Press for helping put it together. I must also give thanks to Scott McGrew for creating such amazing maps, and to Susan Haynes, who shared my vision of this book and played a huge part in bringing that vision to fruition.

When you're researching a book about sea kayaking, having a great boat to paddle is a must. Fortunately, Jim Koehler from the Dinghy Shop provided me with just such a boat and saw that it remained in excellent condition. Knowing where to paddle that boat is yet another requirement. For that expertise I can thank Ray Clarkson, who shared with me his list of favorite kayaking places; Bonnie Aldinger and the crew from the Sebago Canoe Club, for taking a day to show me around Jamaica Bay; and Raymond Howell of the Gowanus Dredgers, who not only provided me a wealth of information about the Gowanus Canal but also opened a fire hydrant so I could rinse off my boat after paddling on

it. Thanks also to Margaret Falk and Travis Beck from the New York Botanical Garden, who escorted me through the construction zone I stumbled into while paddling the Bronx River and gave me an impromptu guided tour of the gardens.

As I was writing the descriptions of the many places I paddled, dozens of questions arose. To find the answers I needed, I often turned to the members of my local paddling club, Long Island Paddlers (**lipaddlers.org**). In particular, Steve Berner offered much advice and, together with Mike Matty, created the system I've used to rate the difficulty of every paddle in this book. Ken Fink, Chris Scalisi, and Nick DeNezzo worked with me during the club's skills days, helping (or at least trying to) make me a better kayaker. And Fred Hosage gave selflessly of his free time to come paddle with me, even though it was getting dark, the tide was dropping quickly, and we would have a current to fight on the way back to our cars. I thank you all for your help, advice, and companionship.

I must also give special thanks to my amazing family for all of their encouragement, generosity, and love throughout the writing of this book. My sister Randy and her husband, Jim, gave up a day on the water to keep me well fed in Montauk, while my niece Caitlin and nephew, Cameron, helped tie up my boat and showed me around a bit of Lake Montauk. My sister

Allison, along with my nieces Sophia and Delaney, helped occupy my own children while I spent many a weekend paddling. And Allison's husband, Eric, provided me with much-needed gear, information, and solutions to problems. All kayakers need someone responsible on land to know their whereabouts and itinerary in case an emergency occurs. Thankfully, Eric became this person for me, and because of him I felt safer and more secure on the water. And my parents, Sue and Doug, continued to do what they do best: encourage, give, guide, and love. They also helped watch my children when I was out kayaking, kept track of where I was paddling, and made sure I was safe. They also fed me whenever I was hungry (and even sometimes when I wasn't). I hope you know how much it all meant to me.

A few family members even trusted me enough to accompany me on some of my trips, making the paddles much more enjoyable in the process. Eric, Allison, Laura Stiegelmaier, and my father tagged along as I paddled everywhere from East Hampton to Staten Island. Remarkably, they never complained when they got muddy, tired, hot, lost, or caught in a thunderstorm. Thank you all for giving of yourselves and your time, and for sharing these experiences with me.

Finally, I have to acknowledge my two children, AnnaGrace and William, whom I love more than anything else in the world. Thank you for your unlimited hugs and kisses, for your love and support, and for always making me smile.

—*Kevin Stiegelmaier*

PREFACE

As someone born and raised on Long Island, I've always felt a strong sense of attachment to this place. Early-morning fishing trips with the family, days at the beach swimming, collecting shells, and watching seals—all helped solidify my love of the island and, of course, its waters. In high school that love led to a scuba certification, and in college it resulted in a degree in marine biology. The purchase of a house near the water was a by-product of it as well. As strange as it may sound, Long Island has played a large role in shaping my life thus far.

With such an affinity for the area, I thought it only logical that after writing a statewide paddling guidebook, *Canoeing & Kayaking New York,* I would eventually write one that focused solely on Long Island. So, after taking some time off to rest (and rinse out my paddling gear), I began researching this new book and planning the many paddles it would include. This process, I assumed, would be much easier than it was with the first book. After all, I was very familiar with Long Island and had been paddling much of its water for years. I soon learned that it was going to take more work than I had thought.

I have my favorite places to paddle and, of course, was planning on including them in the book. But before I got too far into my research, I also wanted to see what places other people enjoyed. So I sent out queries to my paddling friends, their friends, and even friends of friends of friends. A few locations stood out right away as popular favorites: Sebonac Creek, Hallock Bay, the Carmans River. Then there were the personal picks, which varied as much as the people naming them. Some folks favored rough, wide-open water like that at Montauk Point; others preferred smaller, more protected spots like West Meadow Creek. Still others were drawn to locations somewhere in between, like Huntington Harbor.

It had become clear to me that Long Island was home to an incredible variety of paddling opportunities with something for everyone. I also realized that I had a daunting task ahead of me—choosing 50 of these amazing spots to write up for the book. Nevertheless, I consulted my charts, read firsthand accounts, drove to put-ins, scouted beaches, and, finally, created my list of what would hopefully be the best of what Long Island has to offer.

As I began to paddle the waters on this list, I found that most of them were just as good as I had hoped. Descriptions of beautiful beaches, lush plant life, amazing wildlife, and scenic water views soon filled my notebooks. Unfortunately, so did assessments like *muddy, bug-infested,* and *unnavigable.* Some days were warm and sunny, others cold and dreary. Calm water seemed to be as common as rough. The birds of summer left in the fall, only to be replaced by the winter denizens. Seals showed up, ice formed and thawed . . . and I paddled through it all.

Four tubes of sunblock, two pairs of neoprene gloves, three pairs of wet-suit booties, two GPS units, and hundreds of miles later, I had kayaked my way across the island and had loved every minute of it. What emerged from all of this was a better understanding of Long Island and its waters, a greater appreciation for its plant and animal life, a deepening of the love I had already felt for the area, and a belief that the 50 places I ultimately chose to include in the book were indeed the best places to kayak on the island.

Of course, these locations vary greatly in length, difficulty, scenery, and type of water. They are a testament to the wide range in ecosystems found on Long Island. Everything from unspoiled harbors on the island's eastern end to the canals of New York City is included in these pages. Among the 50 paddles are trips in the rivers of the Pine Barrens, by the islands in the center of Peconic Bay, and alongside sandy beaches on the island's South Shore.

As you read about the places in this book and begin to plan your own paddling trips on Long Island and on into the waterways among the boroughs of New York City, remember that what I've written is meant only as a guide. I spent a good deal of time researching put-ins, tide levels, average sea conditions, and potential water hazards so you don't have to. I also described a trip on each body of water that would, in my opinion, showcase the best of what it had to offer. Does this mean you must follow my directions verbatim? Absolutely not. Part of the joy of sea kayaking is exploring new places and creating your own adventures. Perhaps for you that means getting lost in a maze of salt-marsh channels. Or maybe it means finding a deserted beach that's the perfect spot for a picnic lunch. It could also mean encountering wildlife that you weren't expecting. Sometimes it's good to plan your own trips. It is my hope that this book will give you a little extra help in doing just that.

RUN RECOMMENDATIONS

As I considered this book's 50 amazing paddles, settling on the best of the best was no easy task. But for the attributes in the eight categories below, the following destinations won out based on my own experience and observation. These sites include freshwater rivers, tidal creeks, bays and harbors, water trails, and a lake. In alphabetical order, the categories are as follows:

BEST BEACHES

1 Accabonac Harbor (*page 18*)
9 Georgica Pond (*page 56*)
17 Mecox Bay (*page 90*)

BEST SCENERY

18 Montauk Point (*page 95*)
29 Sebonac Creek (*page 141*)
50 New York Upper Bay (*page 235*)

BEST FOR FISHING

18 Montauk Point (*page 95*)
47 Jamaica Bay (*page 222*)
48 Little Neck Bay (*page 227*)

BEST FOR SECLUSION

11 Hallock Bay (*page 64*)
18 Montauk Point (*page 95*)
27 Robins Island (*page 134*)

BEST GEOLOGIC SITES

15 Lloyd Harbor (*page 80*)
18 Montauk Point (*page 95*)
38 Hempstead Harbor (*page 182*)

BEST WATER TRAILS

4 Coecles Harbor
Marine Water Trail (*page 34*)
New York City Water Trail
(*includes all paddles in Part Three*)

BEST FOR KIDS

3 Carmans River (Upper) (*page 29*)
36 West Meadow Creek (*page 171*)
41 Norman J. Levy Park, Merrick
(*page 195*)

BEST FOR WILDLIFE

18 Montauk Point (*page 95*)
35 Three Mile Harbor (*page 168*)
47 Jamaica Bay (*page 222*)

USING THIS GUIDE

This guidebook provides all the essential information you need to plan the paddling routes described. For each route you will learn about the waterway's location, size, history, and typical wildlife. A locator map, trip description, and at-a-glance key information will come in handy from start to finish on each paddling trip. GPS coordinates for put-ins, take-outs, and tide stations, U.S. Geological Survey (USGS) quadrangles, trip length, optimal paddling conditions, mean monthly water temperatures (where available), shuttle directions, and tide information are among the many crucial pieces of information included.

THE MAPS

✧ THE OVERVIEW MAP AND OVERVIEW-MAP KEY

Use the overview map on the inside front cover to find the exact locations of each paddle's put-in/take-out. Each paddle's number appears on the overview map, on the map key facing the overview map, and in the table of contents.

✧ REGIONAL MAPS

This book is divided into three regional sections—Suffolk County, Nassau County, and New York City—and prefacing each section is an overview map of that region. The regional map provides more detail than the overview map, bringing you closer to the hike.

✧ PADDLE MAPS

Detailed maps show the most common and convenient put-ins/take-outs, and they identify points of interest such as bridges, parks, side channels, islands, and marinas. While these maps are extremely helpful in navigating each body of water, I recommend using them in tandem with more-detailed maps. Examples include DeLorme's state-by-state *Atlas & Gazetteer* series (**delorme.com**) and true nautical charts printed by the National Oceanic and Atmospheric Administration (**nauticalcharts.noaa.gov**). Such charts are also stocked at most boating-supply stores, offered as free printable booklets (**ocsdata.ncd.noaa.gov/BookletChart**), and available by subscription at **Trails.com.**

✧ LEGEND

A key to the symbols found on all maps appears on the inside back cover.

RUN PROFILES EXPLAINED

Each paddle trip's profile includes the following elements:

◇ OVERVIEW

These introductory remarks typically cover the body of water's most common put-in and take-out spots; points of interest along the way; the history of the waterway and its surrounding areas; flora and fauna that typically can be observed from a kayak throughout the year; and other features such as beaches, inlets, marinas and mooring fields, portages, rest spots, and side trips.

◇ KEY INFO

Here, nine specifics are cited for each route: its trip level, distance, time, navigable months, potential hazards, number of portages, easy-to-difficult rescue access, tidal conditions, and scenery rating.

Trip level indicates expected paddling difficulty based on possible wind strength, wave size, current speed, and other variables that take place on open water. In this guide, a rating system on a scale of 1–5, developed by members of Long Island Paddlers, determines the levels shown with each entry:

Level 1 indicates a trip on protected waters with few, if any, waves; light to no breeze (less than 10 mph); and no current.

Level 2 alerts you to stronger winds (10–15 mph), waves of up to 2 feet, and a slight current.

Level 3 signals that 2- to 3-foot waves are likely, as are winds up to 20 mph, currents of 3–4 knots, and potential open-water crossings of up to 5 miles long.

Level 4 trips may have longer crossings of up to 10 miles long, currents stronger than 4 knots, 3-foot (or higher) swells, winds up to 20 mph, and difficult landing conditions.

Level 5 denotes open-water crossings of potentially more than 10 miles, large swells, challenging surf conditions, strong currents with turbulence, and waves higher than 4 feet. Winds may be quite strong, and landings could be very difficult.

The Long Island Paddlers rating system also acknowledges trip durations and distances, using a letter between A and D following the level number:

A indicates a short trip, less than 3 hours and 6 miles long.

B denotes a trip lasting 3–5 hours and running 6–10 miles long.

C trips last 5–6 hours and run 10–15 miles, with few places to stop and rest.

D trips require more than 6 hours of paddling and run more than 15 miles, with very few landing spots.

Distance is listed in miles, from put-in to take-out. The distances of side trips, optional paddles, and alternative put-ins or take-outs are addressed in the Description. The average **time** for each trip is listed in hours. These times are meant only as guidelines, however, and can change depending on how many breaks, lunch stops, or photo opportunities you take. **Navigable months** lets you know when conditions are typically and most consistently best for paddling a given body of water. (Of course, many places can be paddled at times other than those listed.)

Hazards comprise such factors as open-water crossings, boat traffic, tidal currents, dams, strainers, deadfall, and waterfalls. Most of these trips require no **portages,** but where applicable the number of them needed is listed in the Key Info.

Ease of **rescue access** is listed according to this scale: *Easy* (rescues can be accomplished throughout an entire trip), *Limited* (rescues can be accomplished at a small number of points during a trip), or *Difficult* (rescues can rarely be accomplished, if at all, throughout a trip).

Tidal conditions refers to the period of time before or after high tide when conditions are best for paddling that route (see page 7 for an in-depth discussion of tides). However, paddlers need not limit themselves to the time spans given, as many bodies of water are at least partially navigable throughout all tidal phases. The paddle route's nearest **tide station,** or sea-level gauge, is listed with its latitude and longitude data, along with the put-in and take-out, in the GPS Coordinates box (see next section).

The last item in the Key Info section, **scenery** is rated on the following scale:

A Beautiful, mostly pristine areas surround the water.

B The area is developed, though still scenic.

C The area is significantly developed.

D The area is extremely over-developed and possibly polluted, and has been stripped of its natural beauty.

✧ GPS COORDINATES

The coordinates of the put-in and take-out spots for each paddle, along with the coordinates for the nearest tide station (where applicable), are provided in latitude–longitude format. In this system, lines of latitude, or *parallels,* run horizontally across the globe, equally distant from each other. Each parallel, expressed in degrees, is roughly equal to 69 miles, although there is a slight variation because the earth is not a perfect circle but an oval. Nevertheless, the equator is considered 0°, while the North Pole is 90°N and the South Pole is 90°S.

Also expressed in degrees, lines of longitude, or *meridians,* run vertically on the globe, perpendicular to latitude lines. Instead of being equidistant, however, they converge at the poles. As a result, they are widest at the equator (about 69 miles apart) and become increasingly narrow as they move north or south. The Prime Meridian, in Greenwich, England, is designated as 0° longitude. From this point, the meridians continue east and west, until they meet 180° later at the International Date Line in the Pacific Ocean.

In this book, latitude–longitude coordinates are expressed in degrees and decimal minutes. For example, the put-in and take-out coordinates for Accabonac Harbor (page 18) are as follows: N41° 01.115' W72° 08.738'; N41° 01.115' W72° 08.738'. These coordinates can also be expressed in degrees, minutes, and seconds. To convert from this format to degrees and decimal minutes, divide the seconds by 60. For more on GPS technology, visit **usgs.gov.**

✧ USGS QUADRANGLES

Probably the most popular, and useful, USGS maps are their 7.5-minute, or 1:24,000-scale series, known as quadrangles. These "quads" provide a good amount of detail and are quite useful for navigation. For this reason, the quads that include particular sections of the bodies of water being described are listed before each Description.

✧ MEAN WATER TEMPERATURES BY MONTH

The USGS maintains hundreds of gauge stations that collect various water data useful to paddlers. Some of these stations take frequent water-temperature readings that can be accessed at **waterdata.usgs.gov/ nwis/rt.** Various private organizations such as fishing clubs, hatcheries, and academic institutions also measure

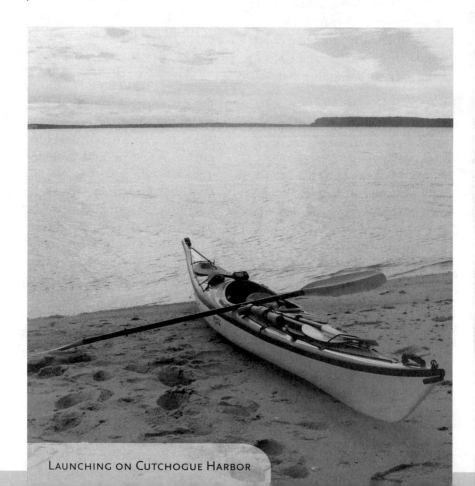

LAUNCHING ON CUTCHOGUE HARBOR

water temperatures. The mean water temperatures are listed by month whenever this data is available.

✧ DESCRIPTION

Here you'll find the play-by-play details of the paddle route for each of the 50 entries in this book. This information is presented so that you could follow it sentence-by-sentence and have an enjoyable journey. You may want to segue to some of the suggested side trips, and you may want to dally or rush: it's all up to you, but this section will guide you from the put-in to the take-out.

✧ SHUTTLE DIRECTIONS

Specific shuttle directions to each put-in and take-out spot are given from a major road or highway. Other shuttling options, such as trains, buses, and subway systems, are also listed wherever possible.

GENERAL SAFETY

HAZARDS

As with most outdoor sports, kayaking is a fairly safe activity, although it does have its share of inherent risks. As such, paddlers should be prepared to encounter any number of the following hazards on the water.

Tidal currents occur whenever an incoming or outgoing tide squeezes through a narrow opening, creating a restricted flow that speeds up the water's velocity. These currents often occur near the mouths of tidal creeks but can also be found near inlets and wherever an island obstructs the normal flow of water. Anytime kayakers

paddle more than a half-mile or so from the shore, or on unprotected water, they are on what is considered to be **open water.** This water is easily influenced by wind and waves, and its conditions can change rapidly. Furthermore, because of the distance from shore, rescues are often difficult to accomplish. Many paddling destinations also make excellent powerboating spots and, as such, often see a good deal of **boat traffic.** This movement of boats most often occurs within marked channels but can also take place within mooring fields and near marinas. **Strainers** are any kind of tree, branch, or other vegetation that is at least partially submerged in a river. The term *strainer* refers to the tendency of such obstacles to allow only water to flow through, trapping everything else in their clutches. **Deadfalls** are similar to strainers but usually block a stream completely and are difficult to get by. There may sometimes be **standing waves,** or waves that do not change position on a river as water flows past them. Depending on weather and prevailing conditions, a river may sometimes overflow its banks, creating **flooding** conditions. Rivers can also flow beneath **tunnels and bridges,** sometimes for long distances. In addition, paddlers may risk **hypothermia/ hyperthermia** and **sunburns.**

RESCUE AND EVACUATION

As stated previously, kayaking carries certain inherent dangers that may not always be avoided. Although such dangers may be slight and may even lead to a more enjoyable experience, they can make paddling a very risky adventure. In fact, times may arise when a boater ends up in such a dire situation that rescue and evacuation are required. Regardless of experience and skill level, all kayakers should be prepared for such circumstances and know how to react should the need arise.

Fortunately, paddlers have many options for minimizing risks and keeping their minds at ease, one of the most important of which is to carry the proper safety equipment. While some items may change as seasons come and go, some basic gear should always be part of every paddler's kit. A properly fitting personal flotation device (PFD) is a must, regardless of weather and water conditions. It's also the law in New York State for paddlers under age 12 or anyone paddling between November 1 and May 1. Appropriate immersion gear should also be worn; a wet suit and dry top may be enough when the water is warm, while a dry suit is highly recommended during cold months.

In addition to a PFD and immersion gear, a paddle float and bilge pump should accompany you on every paddling trip, as should a spare paddle and a noisemaking device such as a whistle or small air horn. I also tuck about 20 feet of parachute cord into the pocket of my PFD and carry a first-aid kit, strobe light, and submersible VHF radio with me anytime I'm on the water. Such items, while not absolutely necessary, are strongly recommended.

A cell phone in a watertight container is also a smart piece of equipment to carry. More-serious outdoorspeople may even choose to carry a personal locator beacon (PLB) or a satellite messenger–GPS tracker. Although these devices cannot be used like a cell phone to call whomever you want, they can be activated to send a distress signal to search-and-rescue groups in the event that help is needed. PLBs and satellite messengers do cost quite a bit of money, though they often are available for rent.

Of course, even the best safety and paddling gear is pointless if you don't know how to use it. Paddlers interested in increasing their knowledge and bettering their skills might consider taking a kayaking class. Such classes are offered throughout the year by many groups across Long Island (see Appendix B) and are usually sponsored by the American Canoe Association. Check **americancanoe.org** for more information.

It's still important to remember that not every body of water is suitable for everyone, even those who are well trained and have a boat packed with safety gear. Paddlers should always keep in mind their abilities and comfort levels when choosing places to kayak. When thinking about paddling a particular bay or harbor, you should consider the length of time needed to complete a trip just as much as the site's level of difficulty. Weather and tidal influences should also weigh heavily in the decision to run or not. A good rule of thumb: "When in doubt, don't go out."

Assuming you've been properly trained and have all of the requisite gear for a safe and enjoyable paddle, the last and perhaps easiest precaution to take is simply to let someone know exactly where you'll be and what your itinerary is. A float plan may prove invaluable in the unlikely event that you run into trouble and need to be rescued. *Sea Kayaker* magazine has created a basic format for such a plan that anyone may use; look for it at **seakayakermag .com/PDFs/float_plan.pdf.**

HELPFUL INFORMATION

TIDES

While many factors determine the conditions on a particular body of water, perhaps none are as important to sea kayakers as the tides. They can make all the difference between a quick and easy trip and a slow and painful slog. They can also open up large areas of navigable water or leave them completely inaccessible. In short, knowing what the tide states are and using that knowledge to help plan your paddles can ensure you of a safe and enjoyable day on the water.

Many variables affect the earth's tides, the most pronounced of which is the gravitational pull of both the sun and moon. Indeed, both heavenly bodies exert this force on the planet and its waters, although lunar pull is more prominent since the moon is much closer to the earth. As a result, it pulls the water on the side of the earth it faces toward itself, creating what we know as a high tide. This leaves less water elsewhere on the planet, otherwise known as a low tide. Amazingly,

the moon also tugs on the far side of the earth, which actually distorts the planet's shape enough to cause another high tide. Thus, there are actually two high and two low tides each day as the earth spins on its axis.

With two of each type of tide occurring each day, one would expect the time period between each high and low to be an equal 6 hours. In fact, the difference is a bit longer—6 hours and 12.5 minutes, to be exact. The reason is that tides are based on a lunar day that lasts 24 hours and 50 minutes, whereas our common solar day lasts only 24 hours.

Another unique feature of this system is the phenomenon of spring and neap tides. *Spring tides* are those that are higher and lower than the normal high and low tides, while *neap tides* show less of a change than is usual for an area. They cycle back and forth about every week, as the positions of the sun and the moon change relative to each other and to the earth. For example, the sun and moon are both aligned with the earth around the time of both a new and full moon, which increases the overall pull of gravity on the earth and its waters and causes spring tides. Likewise, the sun and moon are at right angles to each other when the moon is at a first quarter or third quarter. They limit each other's effect on the earth's waters at these times, thus causing a neap tide.

There is one more piece of the tidal puzzle that may be just as important as knowing what causes high or low tides: paddlers should understand how the changing tides and their currents interact with the environment around them. For example, as a tide rises or falls, water will flow into or out of an area, flooding or ebbing, respectively. As it does this, it may get pinched between two land masses or pass over a deeper region of water, speeding up the tidal current as a result. Alternately, currents running through a wider gap in land masses or over shallower water will slow down. Tidal currents can also form reverse eddies, or areas where the flow actually heads in the opposite direction, wherever they pass an obstruction such as a jetty, dock, or sandbar. As anyone who has ever tried to paddle against a strong current can attest, reverse eddies can be a blessing.

Obviously, the tidal system is very complex and would be quite hard to keep track of were it not for tide tables. A paddler's best friend, these charts predict the heights and times of both high and low tides, sometimes listing the information years in advance. Tide tables can be found in most major newspapers and are also printed in convenient booklets sold in boating-supply stores. They are also published annually in the legendary *Eldridge Tide and Pilot Book* (to order, call 800-992-3045 or 617-482-8460) and are updated continuously on websites such as **saltwatertides.com** and **mobilegeographics.com.** If you own a smartphone, you can even download apps that literally put tidal information in the palm of your hand.

WEATHER BY SEASON

✧ WINTER

Long Island experiences relatively mild winters, with average temperatures around 31°F. Along with New York City, it may only see temperatures fall below zero in two or three winters a decade. Such conditions are due in part to these locations' proximity to water. The Atlantic Ocean, Long Island Sound, and Great South Bay retain their summer warmth for quite some time and warm the land near them as a result. Long Island's winters aren't overly cold, but they are usually quite wet, with about 3.5 inches of rain and anywhere from 3–10 inches of snow falling each month (although some parts of the island may receive more precipitation than others).

✧ SUMMER

Moderately high temperatures are usually seen on Long Island and in New York City during the summer months. These areas are also considerably more humid than other areas of the state because of their proximity to large bodies of water. Thankfully, these waters also bring breezes to the island most summer afternoons, making the heat more bearable.

Summer also marks the beginning of Long Island's hurricane season, with storms most likely to hit during August and September. Some incredibly strong hurricanes have hit Long Island in the past, leaving behind significant damage and greatly altering the island's topography. Fortunately for its residents, Long Island sits at a high enough latitude with cold enough waters that most storms weaken before they strike. Nevertheless, hurricanes remain a potential danger during the warm, humid dog days of summer.

⟡ SPRING AND FALL

Long Island's weather is quite pleasant during these seasons, again because of the moderating effect of the Atlantic Ocean, Long Island Sound, and Great South Bay. Because these waters warm slowly during the spring, they cool the air considerably, keeping the island's temperatures in the 60s until mid-May. Conversely, these bodies of water retain their summer heat and help warm the land near them. Thus, Long Island can see temperatures hovering in the 70s throughout much of September and October.

WILDLIFE

⟡ INSECTS

While Long Island has no dangerous native insects, there are three that can cause a great deal of discomfort and annoyance: the mosquito, the greenhead fly, and the tick.

All three, unfortunately, are plentiful across Long Island and the New York City area, although mosquitoes and greenheads are predominantly found along the beaches and marshes of both the North and South shores. Both are incredibly aggressive biters and cause welts that burn and itch. They often occur in swarms that have been known to follow a person for long distances. These species are most active during spring and early summer months, although both pests can sometimes remain active well into the fall. Dozens of repellents exist; everyone has a personal favorite. The most common comprise a bug net that can be worn over the head and bug spray. Most people agree that sprays containing DEET work the best, although there is some evidence that the chemical can lead to certain health problems. Organic sprays sometimes work just as well as the others. Keep in mind that different repellents may work for different people, so try a few and find the one that works best for you.

Ticks, on the other hand, are tiny parasitic arachnids that live by feeding on the blood of other animals. Two distinct species—the wood (dog) tick and its smaller cousin, the deer tick—can be found on most parts of Long Island but are most prevalent inland near its center and farther east on both the North and South forks. While both kinds of ticks are a nuisance, the tiny deer tick is the one to be most wary of, as it has been found to carry and transmit Lyme disease. In general, deer ticks are much smaller than wood ticks—about the size of a freckle—and are uniformly dark in color, whereas wood ticks usually have white spots.

Though ticks pose little threat to paddlers on the water, they can easily catch a ride on your clothing or gear while you're walking from your car to the shore, or while you portage or camp. The best way to prevent picking up these unwanted tagalongs is to wear long pants and long-sleeved shirts in light colors, so the pests are easy to spot and remove. Bug repellent also keeps them away. Once off the water, thoroughly check your arms, legs, hair, and the rest of your body for any attached ticks. For ticks that are already embedded, removal with sharp tweezers is best: place them as close to skin as possible and gently rotate out, taking care not to squeeze the tick. Use disinfectant solution on the wound.

Although it takes a few hours for a tick to transmit a disease to a person it's bitten, the site should be watched carefully for the next few days for any changes. Lyme disease often shows itself as a red, circular, bull's-eye-shaped rash, but it may not produce any outward symptoms at all. When in doubt, see your doctor.

✧ JELLYFISH

Long Island's waters are home to two species of jellyfish: the moon jelly and the lion's mane (red jelly). While the disk-shaped moon jelly is harmless, the orange lion's mane can produce an itching, burning rash when it stings bare skin. A lion's-mane sting can be serious for a person who is allergic to the venom; otherwise it causes only temporary discomfort. Pouring vinegar on the sting site can alleviate the burning and itching.

✧ REPTILES

The only reptile that may be of concern to Long Island paddlers is the snapping turtle. This fairly large turtle can be found across Long Island in both fresh and salt water. While it usually steers clear of humans, it will bite if disturbed. And with its sharp, hard, beaklike mouth, the snapping turtle can do a lot of damage. Give it a wide berth and it should leave you alone.

CAMPING

Many paddlers often find camping an enjoyable, less expensive, and more convenient alternative to staying in a hotel or inn. Luckily for them, Long

Island has some excellent spots where paddlers can pitch their tents and throw down their sleeping bags.

Two private campgrounds sit on Long Island's North Fork, and a few more lie just beyond the New York City area. These facilities, and more, are listed at **nycampgrounds.com.** Three state parks on the island—**Heckscher, Hither Hills,** and **Wildwood**—also allow camping. Their specific information and reservation details can be found at **nysparks.com/parks.** Finally, both Nassau and Suffolk counties maintain 13 campgrounds in all, widely scattered across the island. The respective counties' websites (**1.usa.gov/ wQpzKl** and **https://parks.suffolk countyny.gov/suffolkcamperweb**) list these sites and provide all the information you might need in planning a stay.

Unfortunately, camping on Long Island is limited to the aforementioned facilities. There are no backcountry areas as in other regions like the Adirondacks or Catskills, where people can set up a tent at no cost. Instead, campers must pay a small fee and stay within a designated space. Nevertheless, camping is a great way to spend time outdoors and lets you experience a side of Long Island that few others have the pleasure of seeing for themselves.

More information about camping in the Empire State can be found in *The Best in Tent Camping: New York State* (Menasha Ridge Press).

NAVIGATIONAL RULES OF THE ROAD

With highly maneuverable boats that are capable of floating on only a few inches of water, we kayakers have the luxury of being able to go almost anywhere. This freedom is likely one of the main reasons people start kayaking in the first place. But because we share the water with other boaters and their wide variety of vessels, it is important to have a working knowledge of the navigational rules and regulations designated by the U.S. Coast Guard. Doing so not only increases your enjoyment of the sport, it helps ensure your safety as well.

As small, human-powered vessels, kayaks have the right of way over larger power and even sail vessels. The latter must yield to paddlers and make sure to not impede their progress. This rule only makes sense when in open water, though, where such vessels can easily change course and speed. Most encounters between kayaks and other boats happen in shallow water, near shore, or perhaps in narrow creeks, channels, or inlets. Under these circumstances, it is the kayaker who is in the more maneuverable boat and, as such, should do whatever he or she can to stay out of other boaters' way.

Besides right of way, kayakers should also be able to recognize common navigational aids and understand what they mean for boaters. The two aids most often encountered on the water are the red and green buoys that mark boat channels. Known sometimes as "green cans" and "red nuns" because of their shapes, these buoys provide a visual clue regarding safe paths around shallow water, sandbars, rocks, reefs, structures, and other obstructions. Boaters must remain between the buoys to ensure safe passage.

Of course, kayakers need not restrict themselves to the boat channel, though times may arise when they must paddle across it. At these times, you should cross the channel via a path that is as close to a right angle as is possible. Obviously, you should also make sure that the way is clear and no boats are heading down the channel in either direction. The easiest way to determine direction of travel in any channel is to remember the saying, "Red, right, returning"—in other words, boats returning to a harbor from the sea will always have the red buoys on their right, or starboard, side. Thus, a boat traveling with the red buoys on its left, or port, side will be heading out to sea.

Things get a bit trickier at night, when navigational aids and other vessels are much harder to see. Luckily, most green and red buoys also display lights in their respective colors, which make them quite easy to find. Powerboats must also display lights—green on the starboard side, red on the port side, and white facing front and back—so their location and direction of travel is easy to determine as well. Should you spy a powerboat showing a green light, you can assume the boat is heading right. A white light in front of the green light indicates that the boat is coming closer to the kayak, whereas a white light behind a green indicates it is traveling farther away. Seeing both a green and red light, on the left and right, respectively, means the powerboat is heading straight toward you.

Kayaks are not required to display any continuously shining lights while on the water, but as Coast Guard regulations state, "Small boats should have ready at hand an electric torch or lighted lantern showing a white light which shall be exhibited in sufficient time to prevent collision." For just this reason, I always carry a small flashlight and wear a headlamp when paddling at night. A quick shine on myself or my kayak makes me easily visible to other boaters and makes us all aware of each others' presence.

Finally, you should be aware of one more rule of the road, although this one remains mostly unwritten: common sense dictates that you should be conscious of other kayakers and boaters on the water. Limit groups to small numbers, remain as quiet and in control as possible, give anglers and other nature-lovers plenty of space, and leave nothing behind but a wake. Finally, respect both public and private property on the water and on land—avoid paddling under private docks or piers, landing on private beaches or in designated swimming areas, or launching from private boat ramps without obtaining permission first.

PARKING AND SECURING VEHICLES

While researching this book, I had the pleasure of visiting just about every part of Long Island and New York City and was able to learn a few things about launching kayaks and parking cars along the way. For instance, I quickly found out that the put-ins that are part of the recently developed New York City Water Trail are some of the most convenient and well-set-up launch sites around. They all sport a safe, easy to use ramp, dock, or

gradually sloping beach and in many cases have picnic tables, grass fields, and nearby parking. Even those spots without their own parking area have street parking very close by. The $15 it costs to use these facilities is, in my opinion, one of the best deals around.

Unfortunately, water access is a bit harder to come by on the rest of Long Island. With most of the shoreline considered private property or lying within a town, county, or state park, the everyday kayaker looking for a good place to put his or her boat in the water may sometimes have to pay in order to do so. Most town parks will usually let both residents and nonresidents park in their lots between Labor Day and Memorial Day. Otherwise, they may charge a nominal fee to nonresidents. Some county parks also charge a small entrance fee. **Green Keys** and **Leisure Passes,** available for purchase in Suffolk County and Nassau County, respectively, allow frequent park-users a chance to save a bit of money by paying an annual fee instead of multiple single-use fees. For more information on Green Keys, log on to **bit.ly/ zhjH8G;** for more information on Leisure Passes, visit **nassaucountyny .gov/agencies/parks/leisure.html.**

You can also launch a kayak on Long Island without paying anything, although finding a place to do so can require a bit of creativity. As stated previously, many parks do not charge fees at all during the off-season. The New York State Department of Environmental Conservation has also constructed numerous launch sites and boat ramps that are open to everyone, free of charge. Paddling outfitters that sit right on the water often welcome the launching of boats from their property, although it's always a good idea to stop inside first and say hello. Then there are the many roads that dead-end at the shore, train stations, and shopping-center parking lots, though you should be sure to check for parking restrictions before leaving your car in any of them.

LONG ISLAND AND ITS WATERS

HISTORY AND GEOLOGY OVERVIEW

Although quite young geologically speaking, Long Island has existed in more or less its present state for more than 10,000 years. Seen from above it resembles a fish, with its head facing west toward Manhattan and its tail fin making up the North and South forks, with Peconic Bay in between. This resemblance is so pronounced that even the Native Americans that settled the island centuries ago took note of it and called their home *Paumanok,* or "fish-shaped." What they could not see, though, were the amazing processes that formed the Long Island that we know today. Indeed, its creation began roughly one million years ago, during the Pleistocene epoch, when global temperatures dropped and the first of many massive glaciers began to form.

As these immense masses of ice form, they constantly melt and refreeze in a cycle that ultimately results in movement, or flow, that

is known as an *advance.* As a glacier advances, it scours the land before it of topsoil, rocks, and pieces of bedrock. With its retreat, the glacier deposits most of this substrate in telltale hill-like or ridgelike formations known as *moraines,* with meltwater rivers and streams cutting paths throughout. As global temperatures rise and fall, a particular glacier may advance and retreat again and again, ultimately changing the topography along its route forever.

Such was the case with Long Island, as a series of glacial advances, known collectively as the Wisconsin Glaciation, covered the land and carved out its basic fish shape. In the end, it was the final two of these advances that produced the most lasting results. One ultimately covered most of Long Island before beginning its retreat and depositing its sediment. As it did, it formed a ridge, called the Ronkonkoma Moraine, which extends along the middle of Long Island from what is now Nassau County down the island's South Fork to Montauk Point. This same glacier then stopped again a bit farther north, creating a second ridge, the Harbor Hill Moraine, which runs from modern-day Brooklyn to Orient Point, forming the island's North Fork.

As this final glacier retreated, it left behind the Long Island of today. The small streams created by the melting ice carried fine silt and sand with them before dropping them in what is known as an outwash plain. This sediment ended up south of the Ronkonkoma Moraine and formed Long Island's relatively flat South Shore with its sandy beaches. On the other hand, the glaciers deposited larger sediment (rocks and pebbles) north of the Harbor Hill Moraine, resulting in the rocky beaches that line the island's North Shore. Then, with the rising of sea levels, water filled in the valley north of Long Island to create Long Island Sound. It also flowed between the two moraines and created Peconic Bay. Finally, it flooded a portion of the South Shore's outwash plain and created the Great South Bay and its system of shallow, protected lagoons.

The glaciers also gouged out large portions of the island's North Shore, forming many of its deep-water harbors like Port Jefferson, Cold Spring, and Hempstead. They left behind huge chunks of ice that eventually melted and formed depressions known as kettle holes (Lake Ronkonkoma is a water-filled kettle hole, or kettle lake). And they carved out streambeds that now carry water from underground springs to Long Island Sound (the Nissequogue River), the Great South Bay (the Connetquot and Carmans rivers), and Peconic Bay (the Peconic River).

Though Long Island is no longer affected by glacial activity, it is still being modified by another force: the ocean. Waves pound its shores, water erodes its bluffs, and currents carry its sediments away, further changing the island's topography. Indeed, Long Island's barrier islands were formed as a result of the ocean's actions and are constantly being shaped and shifted. New inlets have formed while existing ones have closed up. Even shorelines have softened and some harbors and bays have shallowed. It's as if the ocean is fine-tuning the work of the glaciers.

LONG ISLAND PADDLING SEASONS

Because of its moderate climate, Long Island is lucky to have a lengthy paddling season. In fact, most of the island's salt water can be paddled year-round, although some sections of its bays and harbors do freeze by late winter. Likewise, the local freshwater rivers—the Upper Carmans, Peconic, and Bronx—often freeze over, as does Lake Ronkonkoma. Unlike the slushy, soft ice associated with salt water, this freshwater ice is quite solid and can often last through February and into March.

Though it means enduring the cold air and water temperatures of winter, paddling along Long Island between December and early March gives kayakers a view to some amazing wildlife. Loons, snowy owls, mergansers, eiders, and dozens of other species of waterfowl come here to spend the winter and can be seen in incredibly large numbers throughout its bays. Seals are also common winter visitors to the island's waters, seen congregating on sandbars and exposed rocks or poking their heads out of the water whenever a kayaker paddles by. Because most of the powerboaters have taken their craft out of the water for the season, paddlers can often have all of Long Island's beauty to themselves.

Conversely, summer on Long Island is an incredibly busy time to be on the water. Powerboaters are back, as are sailors, Jet Skiers,

windsurfers, and kiteboarders. Everyone wants a chance to enjoy the area's
incredible waters for themselves.
Luckily, there is usually more than
enough water for everyone, including
kayakers, to find a place of their own.
And with water temperatures remaining quite warm well into October,
there's more than enough time to
spend enjoying it.

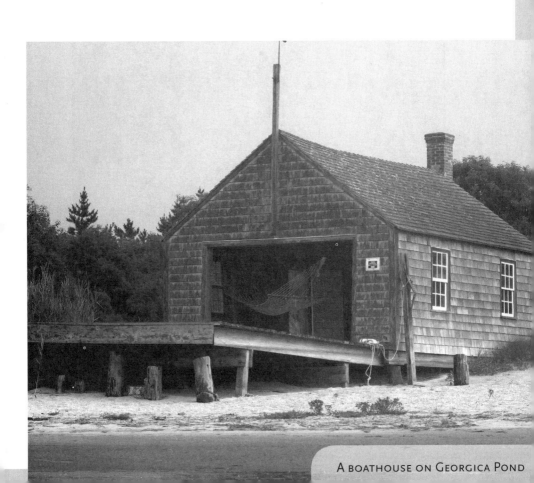

A BOATHOUSE ON GEORGICA POND

Suffolk County (Paddles 1–36)

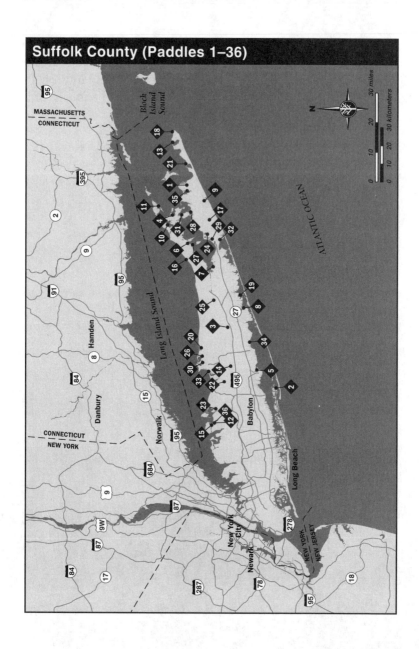

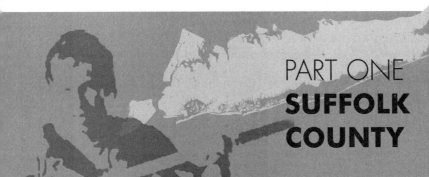

PART ONE
SUFFOLK COUNTY

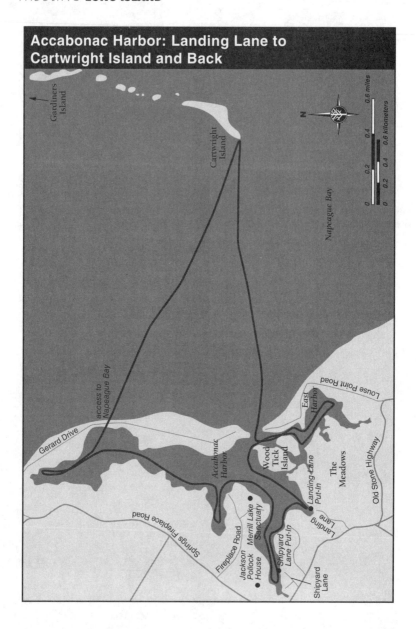

Accabonac Harbor: Landing Lane to Cartwright Island and Back

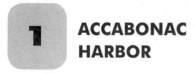

1   ACCABONAC HARBOR

✧ **OVERVIEW** Ask any group of paddlers on Long Island to name their favorite place to paddle, and, if they've ever been there, most of them will say Accabonac Harbor. And rightly so. This small harbor has a lot that makes it such a special place.

First and foremost are its miles of undeveloped shoreline. Though just a short distance from the heart of East Hampton, in a fairly populated part of town known as Springs, Accabonac somehow has managed to evade extensive development. Instead of encountering large waterfront homes replete with Adirondack chairs, barbecues, and boats tied up at docks, visitors to the harbor are greeted by an extensive salt-marsh ecosystem, complete with the usual wildlife species that call such areas home. Accabonac's serene waters flow along low-lying grassy islands, through strands of spartina marsh, and within the mazes of channels in between. The beautiful sandy beaches separating the harbor from the bay are perfect for a short rest, a quick swim, or a long and lazy picnic lunch.

But none of the features that make the harbor so amazing would mean anything if it were inaccessible to paddlers. Thankfully, this is not the case, as two excellent launch sites exist at the end of Landing Lane and Shipyard Lane, respectively. Although neither location boasts more than a safe place to launch a kayak and parking spaces for a handful of cars, both put you on the water—in the southern portion of the harbor—primed and ready to paddle. So while not just anyone can be considered a "Bonacker," as a local is affectionately known, everyone can—and should—come and experience Accabonac Harbor for themselves.

USGS Quadrangles
GARDINERS ISLAND WEST (NY), GARDINERS ISLAND EAST (NY)

1 DESCRIPTION The beauty of Accabonac Harbor is obvious, even if

Landing Lane to Cartwright Island and Back

Level	1B
Distance	8.7 miles round-trip
Time	4 hours
Navigable months	Year-round
Hazards	Open water
Portages	None
Rescue access	Easy
Tidal conditions	3 hours before or after high tide
Scenery	A+

you're just sitting on the beach at the end of Landing Lane. From here, only a small cluster of homes is visible in the distance, with an amazingly vast salt marsh spreading out everywhere in between. Though breathtaking from the sand, this view should be enough to make you jump into your boat as quickly as possible and hit the water.

Once you've launched, paddling out of the small cove and hugging the left (west) shore will bring you to a secluded stretch of water. Here you'll see a handful of homes on the southern shore and the Merrill Lake Sanctuary on the northern side. The latter, owned by The Nature Conservancy, houses one of the most beautiful sections of

GPS COORDINATES

Put-in/take-out
N41° 01.115' W72° 08.738'
Tide station
Promised Land, Napeague Bay, NY
N40° 59.898' W72° 04.902'

marsh on Long Island. It serves as an important habitat for many juvenile fish and marine invertebrates while also providing a home for ospreys, terns, and many species of waterfowl. Stay alert while paddling along its shores, and you may be lucky enough to spy willets, black-bellied plovers, or even a glossy ibis or two.

Besides observing the conservancy property, you can also check out another remarkable landmark within this small stretch of water. The home of abstract painter Jackson Pollock sits in the northeasternmost corner, albeit a bit far back from the water's edge. Heading up the small creek present there during high tides may allow you to get close enough to get a good view of the modest but historic residence.

Head back out onto the main body of the harbor, and you'll see Wood Tick Island to the east. If you look beyond

the island as you pass its northern tip, the harbor's inlet should come into view. Paddling out the inlet will bring you into Napeague Bay, with Gardiners Island and its smaller sibling, Cartwright, off in the distance. On calm days, the crossing to Cartwright can be a pleasant side trip, though it seems a shame to head out onto the bay from here without first exploring Accabonac Harbor's relatively unspoiled northern reaches.

Looking north from the Merrill Lake Sanctuary, the scattering of houses along the narrow causeway to the east will be visible, as will what appears to be a long, unbroken stretch of salt marsh to the west. Study the area using Google Earth, though, and the vast network of mosquito ditches that break up the marsh will also be evident. These ditches were dug, like those in 90 percent of the marshes along the East Coast, to promote a

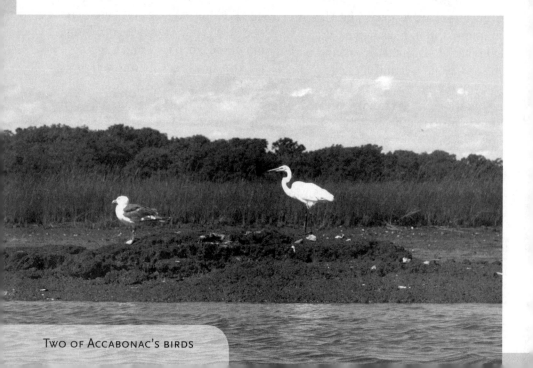

TWO OF ACCABONAC'S BIRDS

greater flow of water into and out of the marsh areas. The thought behind this was that mosquitoes rely on standing water to lay eggs and produce larvae. Thus, if water could be kept from standing, the insects could be kept from laying eggs, effectively stopping the spread of these nuisance critters and the sicknesses they carry.

Although the effectiveness of the ditches is arguable, their detrimental effects on ecosystems have become widely known—they've been found to increased the flow of both pollutants into marsh areas and desirable nutrients out of them. For these reasons, many conservation groups, The Nature Conservancy included, have recently begun taking steps to remedy this problem.

Look up the ditches you'll pass while paddling north along Accabonac's western shore, and you'll see one such effort. Small dams made of sandbags and branches have been erected at the ends of many ditches, slowing down the flow of water and allowing it to remain in the marsh during low tide. This may allow more mosquito larvae to survive in the area, but it also gives predatory fish greater access to the juvenile insects. Unfortunately, these makeshift dams require constant upkeep if expected to continue functioning. Witnessing the breakdown of some of the dams makes it obvious that the conservation groups have a long road ahead of them.

You can paddle more than 1 mile north along this marsh before you reach the harbor's northern tip. Only a few houses, set back a bit from the water, can be seen along the way,

allowing you to focus instead on the large groups of diving terns, swimming cormorants, and wading bitterns and egrets that are quite common here in the spring and summer. Once you've reached the harbor's end, turn around and head south; just 0.5 mile ahead, a narrow bridge provides another access point to Napeague Bay and Gardiners Island, 2 miles distant.

All of Gardiners Island is private property and, as such, is off-limits for boaters. That said, it still makes for an excellent paddling destination, especially the last little piece of land along its southward-stretching archipelago known as Cartwright Island. With an isolated location, a lack of predators, and an abundant supply of food, Cartwright has become home to an astonishing assortment of birds ranging from oystercatchers to terns and black skimmers. Binoculars and cameras are a must for anyone making the crossing. The 2-mile trip should be attempted only during optimal weather conditions, however, as the wind, waves, and tidal currents here can all combine to make the crossing quite dangerous. Remember, too, that landing on the island is prohibited. It is a great spot to observe nature, but not to stop and have a quick bite to eat.

Heading almost due west from Cartwright will bring you back to the mainland and Accabonac Harbor's inlet. This opening can be quite shallow, especially during low tides, and can be crowded with swimmers during hot summer days. Stick to its right (north) side, though, and you should be able to slip through with little trouble. Once you're back in the harbor, Wood Tick

Island will lie directly ahead, with the beach on Landing Lane just beyond that. You may opt to turn left (south) here rather than head back to your car, though, as long as the tide is high enough to allow passage. While nothing more than a mudflat at low tide, this section of the harbor, known as East Harbor, is completely undeveloped and provides another 1.5 miles of shoreline to explore. Just pass around Louse Point, on the inlet's southern shore, head beyond the small flotilla of working boats floating at their moorings, and the area's serenity will be yours.

Just as it will be easy to lose yourself in your surroundings, it may be easy to lose your way back to your put-in. Should this happen, heading back to Wood Tick Island is the best way to

find an open route to the beach. Skirt around the island to the left and you should see the beach at Landing Lane a few paddle strokes later.

✧ **SHUTTLE DIRECTIONS** To get to the put-in at the end of Landing Lane, take NY 27 (Montauk Highway) into the town of East Hampton. Continue heading through town on NY 27 until North Main Street branches off just south of the large windmill. Head north on North Main Street 0.3 mile before turning right onto Accabonac Road. Continue north on Accabonac Road 3.6 miles until it ends. Turn left onto Old Stone Highway and take your first right onto Landing Lane. Look for the small beach and parking area at the road's end.

....

2 CAPTREE STATE PARK

✧ **OVERVIEW** Captree State Park is at the eastern tip of the long barrier island known as Jones Island. Glance at its location on any map or nautical chart, and it's easy to figure out why the park is often described as a fisherman's haven. With the Fire Island Inlet and Atlantic Ocean to the south, a state boat channel to the north, and the whole of the Great South Bay to the east, Captree sits right in the center of some of the best fishing grounds in the northeast. In fact, the park's boat basin is home to the biggest fishing fleet on Long Island.

While most people come here to fish for fluke, flounder, blackfish, and bass, some come to scuba-dive or take a sightseeing cruise. Still others come to make use of the park's beautiful picnic areas, playground, snack bar, and seasonal restaurant. While kayakers do enjoy a good meal, we also take pleasure in paddling through areas with plentiful wildlife. Thankfully, Captree has this to share as well.

Again because of its location, Captree and its surrounding waters are home to many species of birds, including common terns, black skimmers, egrets, herons, bitterns, and even an errant pelican or two. Black ducks are quite common, while loons, long-tailed ducks, and mergansers frequent the area during fall and

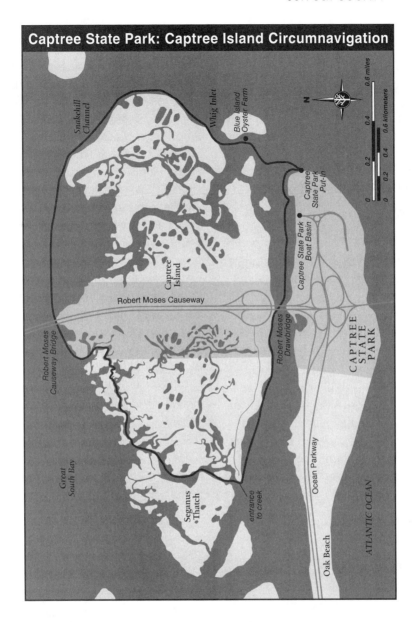

Captree State Park: Captree Island Circumnavigation

Snakehill Channel

Whig Inlet

Blue Island Oyster Farm

Captree State Park Put-In

Captree State Park Boat Basin

Captree Island

Robert Moses Causeway

Robert Moses Causeway Bridge

Robert Moses Drawbridge

CAPTREE STATE PARK

Great South Bay

Seganus Thatch

entrance to creek

Ocean Parkway

Oak Beach

ATLANTIC OCEAN

0.6 miles
0.4
0.2
0
0.6 kilometers
0.4
0.2
0

N

winter months. Blue and horseshoe crabs live here in large numbers, as do many species of bivalves, including clams and mussels. With Captree's proximity to the ocean and its northeast-flowing Gulf Stream current, a few random species of tropical fish can even be found in its waters whenever the current moves close enough to the eastern coast to carry these species far from home.

Although its scenery and wildlife are nothing short of amazing, Captree State Park may not be the best paddling location for everyone. Its waters can be quite busy with boat traffic, its tidal currents can be tricky to navigate, and its fishermen can be hard to avoid. Although such conditions may prove to be little more than nuisances to experienced paddlers, they can be quite dangerous to novices. But when conditions are right, Captree is the ideal place to spend a day on the beach or on the water. Come with your fishing pole, beach chair, binoculars, and of course your kayak and paddle, and enjoy all that it has to offer.

USGS Quadrangles BAY SHORE WEST (NY), BAY SHORE EAST (NY)

2 **DESCRIPTION** Paddling around Captree Island is one of those trips that take a bit of extra work just to begin. The extra work in this case involves paddling a short distance to the north, past the state park's popular fishing pier and across a busy boat channel before finally reaching the island's southern side. But ask anyone who's ever paddled here if this small amount of effort is worth it, and they'll answer with an emphatic "Yes!"

Once you're across the channel and just off Captree's shore, your circumnavigation can begin. The question of whether to round it clockwise or counterclockwise can best be answered by the tide state. You could ride an incoming tide along the island's south shore and paddle around the island clockwise, although you might find yourself fighting the current a bit as you round the eastern side of Captree. Alternately, you could paddle counterclockwise around the island and use an outgoing tide to carry you the last few miles as you head back to the park. Either option is fine, and just as enjoyable as its alternate.

Should you find yourself setting off clockwise, you'll immediately notice that the shore you're paddling along is completely undeveloped. Instead of docks and houses, the scenery comprises little more than a narrow strip of sand with a bit of beach grass beyond, overlooked by a few small trees wherever the land is high enough to remain consistently dry. Look south across the channel or west down its length, though, and you'll see that things are a bit different. The docks that are home to Captree's charter-boat fleet are due south, while a drawbridge spans the channel straight ahead. You'll be paddling the next 1.5 miles between Captree State Park and Captree Island, passing the charter boats

Captree Island Circumnavigation

Level	2B
Distance	5.8 miles around
Time	3 hours
Navigable months	Year-round
Hazards	Tidal currents, boat traffic
Portages	None
Rescue access	Limited
Tidal conditions	2 hours before or after high tide
Scenery	A

GPS COORDINATES

Put-in/take-out
N40° 38.490' W73° 14.905'
Tide station
Oak Beach, NY
N40° 37.998' W73° 16.998'

and under the bridge. The potential danger here lies in the heavy powerboat traffic that will be sharing the water with you. But rest assured: there's enough room for a kayak outside of the channel markers to keep you safe, secure, and out of everyone else's way.

After 0.5 mile you'll come to the drawbridge, which is best navigated on the far right-hand (northern) side. Then, 0.2 mile later, an eclectic collection of waterfront homes begins on Captree's southern shore. Ranging from small shacks to multilevel mini-mansions, almost all of these houses sport a dock of some sort containing any combination of personal watercraft, fishing boats, yachts, and speedboats. This is an excellent spot for doing a bit of people-watching while you paddle past the various setups. The last of these houses comes 0.6 mile later. You can then continue west for another 0.5 mile along Captree's southern shore before you turn the

bow of your kayak north. Alternatively, you can head up the channel just after the last house and bypass the island's southwestern corner altogether. Amazingly, once you make this turn, you'll feel as if you're paddling in a completely different place.

When you examine the island's topography using Google Earth, it's easy to see that there is little difference between water and land within the vast marsh that makes up Captree's interior. Whatever land exists is composed of clumps of peat and banks of mussels. On top of that grows spartina grass, with other marsh plants like phragmites, glasswort, and marsh elder growing a bit higher up. (*Higher up* is a relative term on Captree, though, as most of the island sits only a foot or two above sea level.)

While most of your attention will likely be focused on the sprawling marsh before you, keep an open eye for the many bird species that also

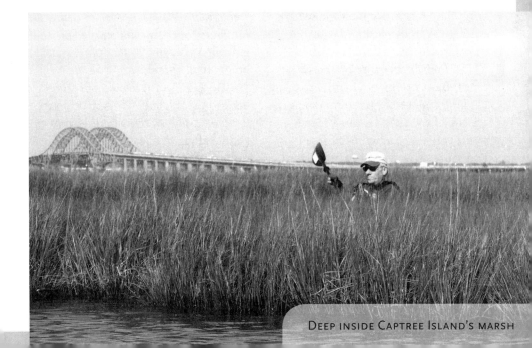

DEEP INSIDE CAPTREE ISLAND'S MARSH

appreciate the island's environment. During spring and summer, the stark white feathers of great egrets will be quite easy to spot as they wade among the green and brown plants of the marsh. Likewise, the aerial antics and dive-bomb fishing techniques of the local terns will be obvious. Harder to spot as it sits almost completely still among the marsh grasses will be the reclusive, extremely well-camouflaged American bittern. Look for its yellow eye and outstretched neck with white and brown stripes. Should you be paddling here during the colder months, large groups of black ducks will appear around almost every corner of the marsh. You also may spy common mergansers, brants, and long-tailed ducks wintering along Captree's shores.

Continue paddling north through the island's marsh, and you'll come to its northern side and gain an excellent view of the Robert Moses Causeway with its iconic arches in 0.5 mile. This is also the time to turn your kayak to the east and continue your circumnavigation along the island's northern shore on the Great South Bay. Alternately, a fairly wide channel cuts through the marsh at the top of the island and also leads to the causeway, albeit in a longer and more meandering manner. In fact, its path is so circuitous that it's easier to carry an overhead image of this stretch of marsh than to try and find your own way through it.

Whichever path you take to the causeway, your next move is simple: pass under it and head around the island's eastern half. From there you can head due south if you want to cut 0.5 mile off the trip. You'll be able to follow the channel that bisects this section of Captree and be back on the island's southern shore in 1.5 miles. Otherwise, head east toward the small, sandy beach 0.6 mile distant if you want to paddle around Captree's entire eastern side.

I recommend taking the latter route, even though it's 0.5 mile longer, as its scenery is quite different from that which you've experienced so far. Unlike the low-lying peat and mussel banks of Captree Island to the west, this side of the island sits on higher and drier ground. As a result, it actually has a fairly wide strip of sandy beach along its length. Because the beach is too dry for the likes of spartina and other saltwater-loving plants, phragmites and poison ivy grow here in abundance. There are even trees growing on this stretch of land, cottonwood and oak being quite prevalent. Unfortunately, the beautiful great egrets that are so frequently seen on the western side are rare here, but you can console yourself with views of willets, sandpipers, and other small shorebirds.

The island's shore starts to curve back to the west about 0.5 mile down its length. Follow this curve as you paddle along the beach, and you'll head toward a narrow gap of water between Captree and an unnamed island to its left. Keep looking as you close the half-mile distance to the break between the two islands, and Captree's only other cluster of buildings should soon appear. Although these houses seem a bit smaller than those west of the drawbridge, they come complete with the same docks and collections of boats as the other cluster.

Once the last of these houses falls astern of your kayak, you'll finally be back on Captree Island's south shore, though there remains one last stop worthy of a visit. Look to the south and you should see a small gray building jutting over the water. This is the home of the Blue Island Oyster Farm, advertised as "the only grower on earth of genuine Blue Point oysters." World-renowned for their taste, Blue Points are named after the region in which they originally grew. In fact, New York State passed a law in 1908 stating that the term could only refer to "oysters that have been cultivated in the waters of the Great South Bay in Suffolk County." Whereas they were once quite abundant in the bay, the Blue Point population has plummeted to endangered levels. Thankfully, with improvements in water quality and conservation efforts by such groups as The Nature Conservancy and local town governments, the oysters have started a comeback.

Once you've gotten a good look at the farm and its bounty, look both ways before crossing the boat channel to the south, then head straight across to the state park and the beach where you began your trip.

◇ **SHUTTLE DIRECTIONS** To get to the put-in at Captree State Park, take the Robert Moses Causeway south and follow the signs for the park. Once there, head toward the easternmost parking lot. Park near the southeasternmost corner and look for the short path that leads to the water's edge.

3 CARMANS RIVER

◇ **OVERVIEW** The Carmans is Long Island's most beautiful and perhaps most protected river. Like all of Long Island's major rivers, it originates from an underground spring, then flows into a series of small ponds in the center of the island. From there it forms a freshwater river, eventually turning into a saltwater estuary that empties into the Great South Bay. Most of the land along its 10-mile length is designated parkland and is almost completely undeveloped. In fact, New York State has designated the Carmans as a Scenic and Recreational River—a distinction that has helped to protect its natural beauty and make it an extremely popular paddling destination.

Although the Carmans flows almost unimpeded from Yaphank to the Great South Bay, most paddlers choose to break it up into two portions: an upper and lower, separated by the dam at the south end of Southaven County Park. Doing so makes perfect sense logistically (the dam's portage can be quite tricky) and geographically (the two sections flow through very different habitats).

The upper, freshwater portion of the Carmans River flows through land

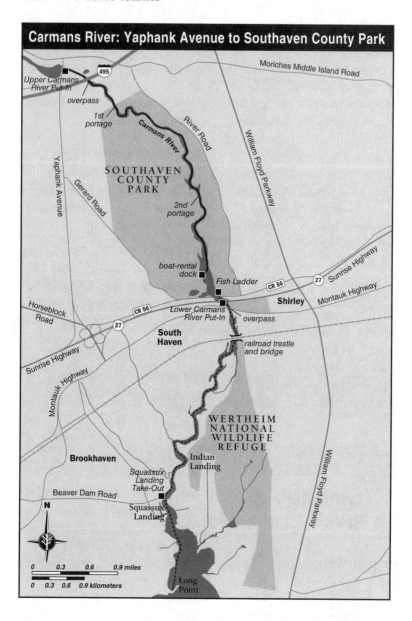

Carmans River: Yaphank Avenue to Southaven County Park

once owned by a hunting and fishing club in the 1800s. In fact, the river— originally known as the Connecticut— was given its present name to pay homage to the operator of the hunting club, Samuel Carman. Thankfully, Suffolk County obtained the land decades ago and forever protected it by creating the 1,500-acre Southaven County Park. Red maple trees abound along this stretch of river, as do pepperidge trees, honeysuckle bushes, swamp rose bushes, and sprawling groves of bright-blue forget-me-nots. Also common are muskrats, brook trout, wood ducks, and cedar waxwings.

The lower, tidal portion of the Carmans River flows just south of NY 27 (Sunrise Highway). Vastly different from the upper river, this estuarine portion lies almost entirely within the bounds of the Wertheim National Wildlife Refuge, a 2,500-acre property designed to help protect the area for migrating birds. Huge stands of phragmites line most of the river in the refuge, augmented by spartina grasses and other salt-tolerant plants. Great blue herons, great egrets, and ospreys are numerous on the Lower Carmans, as are bluefish and striped bass. More recently, a pair of bald eagles has also been spotted on refuge property.

It seems a shame that the river flows through such beautiful and pristine lands, yet access to its waters is either somewhat limited or completely prohibited altogether. Southaven County Park does allow paddling through its boundaries, but only later in the week and for a fee of $2. On the lower river, there is only one convenient spot to put in, on Montauk Highway. Likewise, Indian Landing and Squassux Landing are the only take-out sites available. The Wertheim refuge prohibits visitors from entering by water. But despite its limited access, the Carmans is a true gem from beginning to end. Many who paddle the river declare it one of the prettiest spots they've paddled on the island.

USGS Quadrangles BELLPORT (NY)

3A **DESCRIPTION** The best place to begin your paddle on the Upper Carmans River is just below Lower Lake in Yaphank. Although the

Yaphank Avenue to Southaven County Park **A**

Level	1A
Distance	3.5 miles one-way
Time	2 hours
Navigable months	February–March (weekends only), May–October (Thursday–Sunday)
Hazards	Deadfall
Portages	2
Rescue access	Easy
Tidal conditions	Spring-fed—not affected by tides
Scenery	A+

paddling is not exactly easy on this stretch of river—the water is very shallow and contains submerged logs and deadfall—the exquisite scenery is well worth the extra effort and care needed to navigate it. Red maple leaves hang low over the river, forming a tunnel of sorts to paddle through, while alder branches fill in most of the gaps left open. Expect to see aquatic plants such as buttonbush, water willow, sweet pepperbush, and arrowhead growing at the river's edge, with muskrat, great blue heron, wood duck, and white-tailed-deer sightings just as common.

As the river winds its way south, it continues to flow through this narrow,

GPS COORDINATES

Put-in
N40° 50.113' W72° 54.971'
Take-out
N40° 48.351' W72° 39.822'

secluded environment until it passes under the Long Island Expressway (I-495) 0.3 mile from the put-in. South of the highway, the river widens a bit, making paddling much easier. The more-open river also gives you the chance to observe the myriad colorful insects (including butterflies, damselflies, and dragonflies) that inhabit the Carmans during spring and summer, as well as the striking plumage of the wood duck during fall. Don't get too wrapped up in insect- or bird-watching,

however, because the river leads to a small waterfall just 0.5 mile from the I-495 overpass. This waterfall is visible directly under the concrete railroad trestle but can be heard much earlier. Daring paddlers may simply head straight over the 2-foot drop, though the more cautious, and perhaps smarter, approach is to land your boat on the right-hand (western) bank before you reach the train trestle. From there you can easily walk your boat over the drop and resume paddling on the other side.

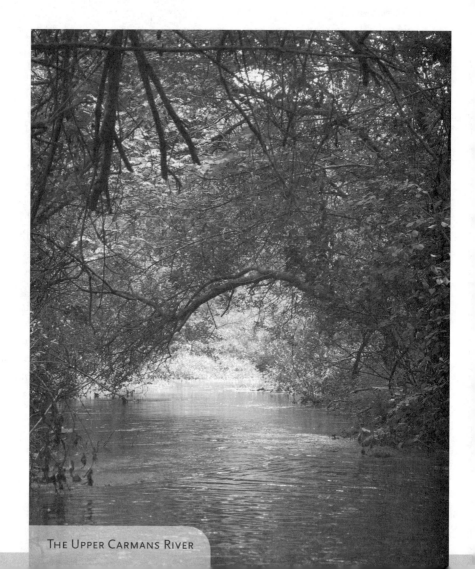

THE UPPER CARMANS RIVER

Once past the waterfall the river widens even more as it enters Southaven County Park. Keep an eye out on land and you should be able to see more pitch-pine trees growing in this new section of river. These trees are known for their resistance to forest fires and are synonymous with the Long Island Pine Barrens region, although they can be found elsewhere across the island. The easiest way to distinguish pitches from other pine trees is by counting the number of needles growing in each bunch: pitch pines will always have three.

The river widens even more past the waterfall, entering Southaven County Park. After 1.5 miles, you'll reach a concrete dam that requires a short portage. Just as with the waterfall, there is a small landing spot on the right-hand (western) riverbank before the dam. Land your boat there and carry it over to the other side of the drop. From this point on, you'll be paddling in the section of the river used by rental boats from the park. The water can get very crowded here, especially on summer weekends. If you stay close to the left (east) riverbank, though, you should be able to avoid most of the boat traffic.

You can end your trip at the rental-boat docks on the right-hand side of the river, in the wide portion known as Hards Lake. You can also continue farther south, paddling the Lower Carmans River to its mouth in Bellport Bay. To do so, you must portage your boat around yet another waterfall. You should be cautious if this is your plan. The current is very swift on the other side of the portage, requiring strength

and care when putting your boat back in the water. A better idea is to paddle to the take-out spot in Southaven County Park and simply drive your boat to the next put-in.

◇ **SHUTTLE DIRECTIONS** To get to the put-in, take the Long Island Expressway (Interstate 495) to Exit 67N (Yaphank Avenue). Turn right onto Yaphank Avenue and travel north about 0.3 mile. You will see the put-in on the east side of the road, across from the Yaphank Lower Lake. You should drop your boat off here but park down the road a bit. To do so, head back the way you came on Yaphank Avenue, taking your first right turn onto Long Island Avenue. There will be a small parking lot on the corner as you turn. Follow the signs and park your car in any available spot.

To get to the take-out from I-495, take Exit 68S (William Floyd Parkway). Travel south on William Floyd Parkway 2.7 miles until you reach Victory Drive. Turn right onto Victory Drive and follow the signs to Southaven County Park and the boat launch.

3B **DESCRIPTION** Unless you're continuing a paddle from the Upper Carmans, the floating dock at the vacant kayak-rental shop on Montauk Highway is the best place to launch on the lower river. You will enter the water just south of the NY 27 (Sunrise Highway) overpass and just north of NY 27A (Montauk Highway). Once you're on the water, the excitement of being there and the immediate beauty of your surroundings may combine

B Montauk Highway to Squassux Landing

Level	1A
Distance	5 miles one-way
Time	2–3 hours
Navigable months	Year-round
Hazards	None
Portages	None
Rescue access	Limited
Tidal conditions	Any
Scenery	A+

to urge you south. Just a short paddle north, however, lies an interesting structure that you may not want to pass by: a fish ladder, designed to help fish like alewives swim upstream. Alewives are anadromous, meaning they spend the majority of their lives in salt water but spawn in fresh water. With a dam effectively separating the upper, fresh-water portion of the Carmans from the lower, marine portion, alewives were long prohibited from returning to their spawning grounds. Thankfully, the fish ladder was installed in 2008, making the alewives' lives much easier.

After turning south and passing under Montauk Highway (NY 27A), you'll be paddling within the borders of Wertheim National Wildlife Refuge.

GPS COORDINATES

Put-in
N40° 48.111' W72° 53.107'
Take-out
N40° 46.440' W72° 53.776'
Tide station
Smith Point Bridge, NY
N40° 44.318' W72° 52.034'

The refuge's headquarters will come into view on the western bank as the river continues south. As it does, a large island will also appear in the center of the river. Both sides of the island are navigable, although the eastern shore is more protected and may give you a better chance of seeing wildlife. The island itself has a slightly barren appearance due to fire. In the spring of 2007, the U.S. Fish and Wildlife Service conducted a controlled burn on the island to rid it of an invasive plant known as phragmites. This plant is known to crowd out naturally occurring plants that are beneficial to local wildlife. While the burn was somewhat successful, it is amazing to see how tenaciously the phragmites has grown back in the three years since.

Past the island, the river takes on a different appearance. Gone are the red maple and birch trees that lined its shores; present in their place are huge stands of cattails and phragmites. If you keep an eye out on the western riverbank for breaks in the reeds, you may discover some side creeks to explore. The northernmost stream, Yaphank Creek, is almost 3 miles south of your put-in. Follow it and you will be led as far north as Montauk Highway. Little Neck Run, another side creek, lies 0.5 mile south of Yaphank Creek. Between these two creeks, on the opposite riverbank, is Indian Landing. This small beach, once a meeting sight for the Unke-chaug Indians, is the perfect spot to beach your boat, have a snack, and stretch your legs. There is also a 0.8-mile nature trail that you can walk in less than an hour.

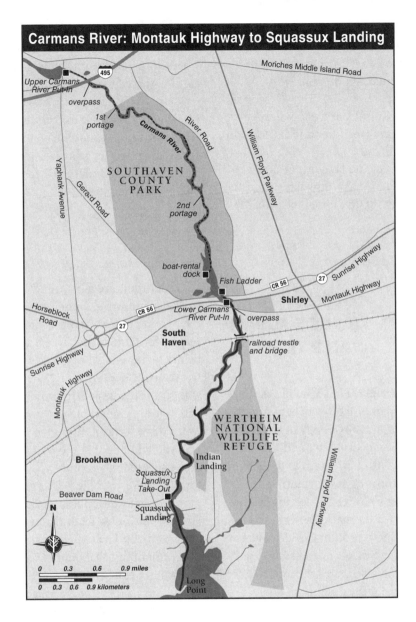

Carmans River: Montauk Highway to Squassux Landing

Many paddlers turn back around after leaving Indian Landing, paddling upstream to the put-in and their cars. The current is usually slow enough to make this easy. Another option, though, is to continue south for another 0.5 mile to the take-out at Squassux Landing. You may also decide to head 1 mile farther downstream to Long Point, the last bit of land before the river drains into the Great South Bay. You will still have to head back to Squassux Landing from there, however, as there is no take-out nearby.

✧ **SHUTTLE DIRECTIONS** To get to the put-in, take NY 27 (Sunrise

Highway) to Exit 58S (William Floyd Parkway). Travel south on William Floyd Parkway, turning right at the second intersection onto NY 27A (Montauk Highway). Stay on Montauk Highway 1 mile, and you will see the vacant kayak outfitter and its dock on your right.

To get to the take-out at Squassux Landing, take Sunrise Highway to Exit 57S (Old Horseblock Road).

Old Horseblock Road will end at Montauk Highway, where you should turn right. Take Montauk Highway until you reach your second left turn, Yaphank Avenue. Yaphank Avenue eventually merges into Old Stump Road and leads you to Beaver Dam Road. Turn left on Beaver Dam Road, and the dock at Squassux Landing will be straight ahead.

4 COECLES HARBOR MARINE WATER TRAIL

✧ **OVERVIEW** Find Shelter Island on any map or nautical chart, and you can't miss the large body of water in its northeast corner, named Coecles Harbor. With Little Ram and Big Ram islands forming its northern boundary and the shores of the amazingly pristine Mashomack Preserve (see page 151) to its south, Coecles Harbor is not only Shelter Island's biggest harbor but also its most protected. Considering the amount of sheltered waters within its confines, you would expect the harbor to be quite popular among the yachting crowd . . . and you'd be absolutely correct. Yet the features that attract an incredible number of large boats during the spring and summer months— namely, the quiet water and scenic shores—also make Coecles Harbor an ideal location for a paddling trail.

Water trails are a hot trend in the sea-kayaking world, popping up all over the country on a variety of waters. The reason for their appeal is best stated by the Water Trails Locator website (**watertrailslocator.com**): "Water trails will give you access to the wilderness with a unique point of view from the water. As you travel through a water trail you will find that the beauty of the area will suddenly capture you, perhaps for the rest of your life." This summary perfectly describes the Coecles Harbor Marine Water Trail, created in 2001 by the local Shelter Island government in collaboration with The Nature Conservancy and Shelter Island Kayak Tours (**kayaksi.com**).

The trail's creators carefully researched and planned a route that brings you effortlessly into the beauty of Coecles Harbor. Paddle its 5-mile length, and you'll float past some modern development and a bit of local history while you also become deeply immersed in the marine environment. Expect to see turtles, fish, waterfowl, and various shorebirds along the trail

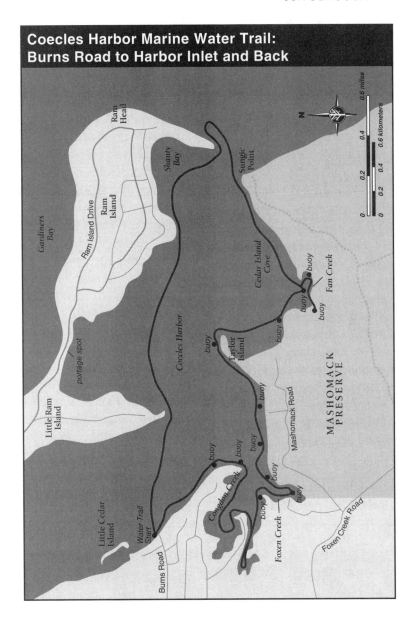

Coecles Harbor Marine Water Trail: Burns Road to Harbor Inlet and Back

and throughout the harbor. You'll also witness the beauty of the pristine, protected salt marshes of The Nature Conservancy's Mashomack Preserve firsthand. You'll likely take dozens of pictures, gaze in awe at your surroundings, and probably learn a thing or two along the way. In short, paddling the Coecles Harbor Marine Water Trail will be some of the most fun you've had in your boat in a long time.

Thankfully, Coecles Harbor is quite easy to access by kayak. More than a few launch sites dot both the north and south shores, although the official start of the trail is at the eastern end of

Burns Road. There you'll find plenty of parking, a small launching ramp, and a kiosk with signs and maps detailing the route. So grab a map, throw your kayak in the water, and head for the first white buoy along the route. There are few better ways to spend a day.

USGS Quadrangles
GREENPORT (NY)

4 **DESCRIPTION** To reach the first stop along the Coecles Harbor Marine Water Trail, head southeast from the Burns Road put-in and hug the shore for a few hundred feet until you reach a small white buoy with a green oak leaf—The Nature Conservancy's logo—painted on top. Like the trail's other buoys, this one floats just 20 feet offshore, making it quite easy to find amid the harbor's dark-green waters. Paddlers may find this buoy's location a bit odd at first, considering its proximity to a well-developed shoreline.

Burns Road to Harbor Inlet and Back

Level	2B
Distance	7.4 miles round-trip
Time	4 hours
Navigable months	Year-round
Hazards	Open water
Portages	None
Rescue access	Limited
Tidal conditions	Any, although some parts may be inaccessible during low tide
Scenery	A+

Nevertheless, the trail's interpretive map identifies this spot as an excellent place to view an example of a shoreline built up with peat mounds and ribbed mussel banks. A quick view to the right (south), especially at low tide, easily confirms this.

By the time you reach the second stop, just 0.5 mile away, almost all the development along the shoreline will be gone, leaving you in an unspoiled environment. From this point, known as Foxen Point, the next buoy is directly across the protected stretch of water called Congdon Creek. Instead of making a beeline for the buoy, though, you may want to head west and explore a bit more of Congdon Creek first. A shoreline of spartina grass, marsh elder, and bayberry bushes set off by oak and cedar trees hugs the creek's northern edge, while its southern branch is a great spot for checking out the small fleet of fishing boats that call its water home. Though only about 0.3 mile long, this portion of the creek can provide a welcome addition to the marine trail if time allows.

Four smaller white buoys forming a square will greet you as you head east out of Congdon Creek and back toward the trail. These other buoys mark the location of one of The Nature

GPS COORDINATES

Put-in/take-out
N41° 04.456' W72° 19.018'
Tide station
Cedar Point, NY
N41° 01.998' W72° 16.002'

Conservancy's shellfish-restoration areas. Such sites have been set up across the entire East End of Long Island in an effort to bring back the clams, oysters, and scallops that once were plentiful in these parts. According to the conservancy, "These protected, no-take zones have concentrated numbers of shellfish, which lead to higher reproductive rates, and more shellfish for the entire area." There's little to see of the operation from the seat of a kayak, but it is encouraging to know that such efforts are under way.

The trail's next two stops lie just a few hundred feet down another small arm of water known as Foxen Creek. More cove than creek, it runs south into the Mashomack Preserve for a short stretch before dead-ending at a wall of vegetation. The trail then leads back out into Coecles Harbor, curving to the northeast toward a unique piece of land called Taylor's Island. Why, you may be asking yourself, is it called an island when it's attached to land? Paddle here during high tide and you may just get your answer, as the sandbar that connects Taylor's Island to Shelter Island is likely to be completely submerged.

As if the "island" designation weren't enough to cause some confusion, Taylor's original name, Cedar Island, may conjure a bit more. Why was it called Cedar Island if there are only a few straggly trees growing on it? Truth be told, an abundance of the species once grew here, although little sits here today but a small log cabin that once belonged to the land's current namesake, S. Gregory Taylor. The cabin is now a registered historic place and Taylor's Island is a town park, open to all paddlers seeking a place to explore, stretch their legs, or enjoy a picnic.

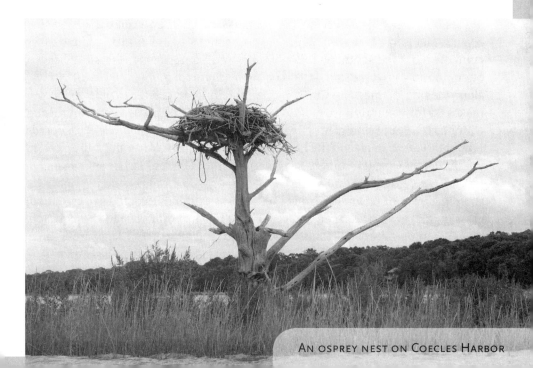

AN OSPREY NEST ON COECLES HARBOR

After you're back on the water, look to the south about 0.5 mile distant and you should see an osprey platform on shore. The trail's tenth stop, just offshore from this platform, appropriately explains the ecological significance of this magnificent bird. Chances are pretty good you'll spot an osprey on this platform or flying nearby, but this wasn't always the case. Osprey numbers declined so precipitously in the late 1960s and the 1970s that the bird was declared an endangered species and thought to be facing extinction. The primary cause, many believe, was repeated ingestion of the pesticide DDT, which weakened the osprey's eggshells. Fortunately, this chemical's use was banned and the bird's numbers began to climb steadily. While they're not out of the woods yet, ospreys are becoming more common along Long Island's marine waterways every day.

After spending some time looking for, and hopefully observing, the ospreys that inhabit the nest on this point of land, head southeast for only 0.2 mile and you'll reach the last creek along the trail. Named Fan Creek, it makes up for its diminutive length with much serenity and natural beauty. Like both Foxen Creek and the northern portion of Congdon Creek, Fan Creek has a completely undisturbed shoreline, brimming with spartina grass, marsh elder, glasswort, and other common salt-marsh plants, surrounded by a forest of oak, maple, and cedar trees. Fan Creek is unlike the other creeks, however, in that all of the previously mentioned plant species border a creek that is only about

10 feet across at its widest point. The quiet, secluded feel this environment gives paddlers is welcoming. It's quite a shame that the creek only runs for a few hundred feet before dead-ending at a line of trees. Thankfully, the last three stops of the trail are along the way, giving you an excuse to paddle slowly and take your time.

Once you've reached the end of the trail, you have a decision to make. If the main focus of your trip was to experience the trail, you may choose to retrace your paddle strokes and make the return trip to the put-in (the most direct route puts it 1 mile away). There is much more to see within the confines of Coecles Harbor's shores, though, and you may want to continue if you have the time. For example, just 0.5 mile beyond the entrance to Fan Creek, along a still-undeveloped shoreline, sits the harbor's inlet. Paddle between Sungic and Reel points, which almost pinch off the inlet, and you'll be floating in Gardiners Bay 9 miles due west of Gardiners Island. While paddling to the island from here is not feasible, heading south for 2 miles to Cedar Point and its lighthouse is a viable option. One may also choose to head north and round both Ram and Little Ram islands before portaging over the causeway and entering Coecles Harbor once again. Finally, some paddlers may simply elect to stay within the confines of the harbor but hug its northern shore, exploring Ram and Little Ram islands from the south side instead. This last option is especially enticing if conditions on Gardiners Bay are not ideal, or if the tidal current racing through the inlet is too much to handle (which it often can be).

Paddling along the harbor's northern shore may take a bit of getting used to, as it is quite different from the southern side. Gone are the nature preserve and its associated unspoiled natural beauty. Here instead are houses and their associated boats and docks. You'll pass more than 2 dozen docks on the southern shore of Ram Island alone. Many of the homes are quite beautiful, however, and can offer just as much enjoyment to the observant paddler as the marine trail did.

As you continue along the bottom of Ram Island, you'll come to a fairly large cove after 1 mile that separates it from Little Ram Island. Keep an open eye and you'll probably see a car or two driving along the causeway that links the islands to the mainland. A few spots along this stretch are suitable for a portage should you want to explore Gardiners Bay a bit. They can make good rest areas for weary paddlers as well.

The gap between the islands can be crossed in just 0.5 mile, bringing you to Neck Point on Little Ram. From there, the start of the marine trail (and your car) is only an additional 0.5 mile away.

✧ **SHUTTLE DIRECTIONS** Take the South Ferry to Shelter Island, continuing north on NY 114 until you reach a traffic circle 1.3 miles later. Head north from this circle on Cartwright Road for 0.75 mile and turn right onto Burns Road. Follow Burns Road to the water, where you can pick up a map of the water trail and launch directly from the beach.

---

5 CONNETQUOT RIVER

✧ **OVERVIEW** Known to Native Americans as "The Great River," the Connetquot is another of Long Island's four major rivers. It originates from a freshwater spring near the center of the island in the town of Islandia. It then flows south for 6 miles, almost entirely within the boundaries of the Connetquot River State Park, before finally emptying into the Great South Bay. Unfortunately, boating of any kind is prohibited on the river while it flows through state-park property. Such a prohibition limits paddlers to the lower, estuarine portion of the river, south of NY 27 (Sunrise Highway).

More limitations exist on the lower portion of the Connetquot. Although paddling on this portion of the river is permitted, access is severely limited. Most of the river's shores are lined with homes and private property. The New York State Department of Environmental Conservation maintains a few fishing-access points near Sunrise Highway but prohibits boat launching from any of them. This leaves paddlers with a single launching site on the Connetquot: Timber Point County Park.

Timber Point's amenities include ample parking, picnic tables, and a sandy beach for launching. In addition, its location, near the mouth of

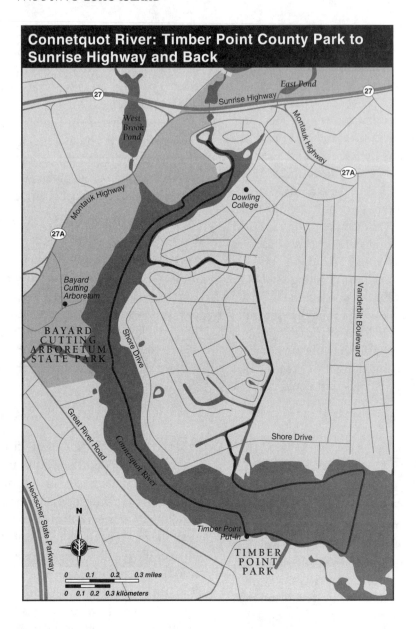

Connetquot River: Timber Point County Park to Sunrise Highway and Back

the Connetquot, puts boaters on the river poised for a trip north toward Sunrise Highway or south to the Great South Bay and Heckscher State Park. Although these are its only two paddling options, the Connetquot has always been, and will likely remain, a local favorite.

USGS Quadrangles
BAY SHORE EAST (NY)

5 **DESCRIPTION** The Connetquot is quite wide near the put-in at Timber Point, with both shores being extensively developed. The eastern shore contains some fairly large boatyards

Timber Point County Park to Sunrise Highway and Back

Level	2A
Distance	6 miles round-trip
Time	3–4 hours
Navigable months	Year-round
Hazards	Boat traffic
Portages	None
Rescue access	Easy
Tidal conditions	Any
Scenery	B–B+

and yacht clubs, while the western shore is lined with houses. Head north along this shore, and these houses eventually give way to a pristine, scenic shoreline 1 mile north of Timber Point. At this point you will reach the Bayard Cutting Arboretum's southernmost boundary. Considering the lack of open space on the river's shores, the natural beauty of the arboretum is welcoming.

Since it was laid out in 1887, this arboretum has, according to its benefactor, Mrs. William Bayard Cutting, served to "provide an oasis of beauty and quiet for the pleasure, rest, and refreshment of those who delight in outdoor beauty." Anyone with time on his or her hands should definitely pay this amazing park a visit. Please note, though, that landing boats is not permitted along the arboretum's

GPS Coordinates

Put-in/take-out
N40° 43.381' W73° 08.863'
Tide station
Great River, Connetquot River, NY
N40° 43.398' W73° 09.102'

shoreline. Its small coves, inlets, and tiny islands are a pleasure to paddle among, however.

After 2 miles, you'll reach the arboretum's northern terminus, where houses dominate the shoreline once again. The Dowling College campus is visible directly across from the river at this point. First a Vanderbilt family mansion, the property was also home to a group of metaphysicians, the site of the National Dairy Research Lab, and part of Adelphi University. Since 1968, it has been known as Dowling College. Lucky paddlers may share the river with Dowling's crew teams as they scull along its length during their workouts.

You'll come to a fork in the river just after the Dowling campus. Here paddlers can head left (west), straight ahead, or right (east). The left branch takes paddlers through a narrow canal lined with private homes before it dead-ends at a low-hanging railroad trestle after about 2,000 feet of paddling. Heading straight or right leads around either side of a small island with a large cedar-shingled house situated firmly in its center. This portion of the Connetquot also dead-ends just south of NY 27 (Sunrise Highway).

After turning around, paddlers may head back to Timber Point County Park the way they came or take a slightly different path, through a canal that joins the eastern shore of the Connetquot 1 mile south of the turnaround. This canal is an excellent place to paddle, especially when you desire a closer, more intimate setting. Waterfront homes and their associated docks and boats line both sides of the passageway, but the water is always still, the people are friendly, the boats move slowly, and the sights are plentiful. With a bit of faith, perseverance, and 0.5 mile of paddle strokes, the houses even disappear, leaving nothing but a quiet and peaceful stretch of water.

A few side channels along the length of the canal can easily be explored should time allow. Otherwise, the canal will empty into the river just 1.5 miles after it starts, directly across from Timber Point County Park. From there, paddlers may head southeast, past the large boat marinas toward the mouth of the Connetquot, or simply due south to reach the take-out. Keep in mind, however, that boat traffic can be quite busy in this portion of the river. Paddlers should take great care when crossing the river and be sure to stay within the boating no-wake zone for ultimate safety.

✧ **SHUTTLE DIRECTIONS** To get to Timber Point County Park, take NY 27 (Sunrise Highway) to Exit 46 (Connetquot Avenue). Head south on Connetquot Avenue 0.75 mile, cross over Montauk Highway, and continue heading south on Great River Road. Look for the entrance to Timber Point County Park after 1.5 miles, just before the road turns sharply to the right.

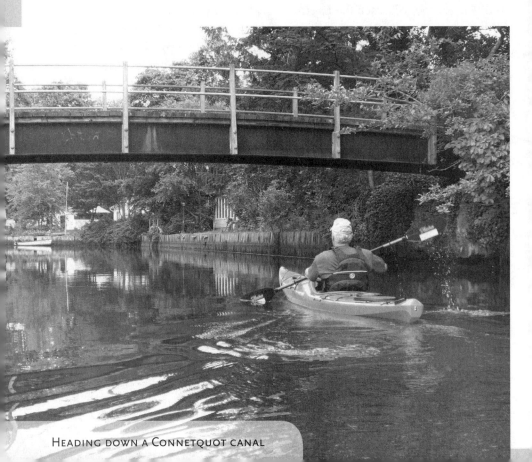

HEADING DOWN A CONNETQUOT CANAL

6 CUTCHOGUE HARBOR

✧ **OVERVIEW** Considered by many, including Albert Einstein, to be one of the most beautiful bodies of water anywhere, Cutchogue Harbor has long been appreciated by both its inhabitants and visitors alike. In fact, the Native Americans who first settled the area in 1000 BC called it *Corchaug*, or "The Principal Place." The land and its abundance obviously meant a lot to these first settlers and their subsequent ancestors, who were motivated to build a large wooden fort to protect the area. Fort Corchaug did serve its original purpose quite well, for the Corchaug people continued living off the land for decades to come, hunting and fishing for what they needed to survive—that is, of course, until 1667, when Europeans arrived from nearby Southold looking to expand their territory.

Hoping to make good use of the area's incredibly fertile soil and bountiful waters, the English staked claims across the Corchaugs' land and set up farms, homesteads, and businesses throughout. These actions apparently sealed Cutchogue's fate, for even now, almost four centuries later, Cutchogue remains a vital center of the North Fork's agricultural community, with vineyards, sod, and produce farms sprawling from one side of the hamlet to the other. Its local business community is still thriving, with many mom-and-pop stores up and down its Main Street. And its harbor has continued to bustle with fishing boats, sailboats, and, more recently, kayaks.

Along with adhering to many of its old ways, Cutchogue has also preserved much of its history in the way of dozens of historic buildings and structures. Most obvious is the "Old House" that sits on the village green. Originally built in 1649 in Southold, the house was deconstructed and moved to its current location in 1661. Thankfully, Fort Corchaug, or what remains of it, has also been protected. Its remnants and 51 acres surrounding them were purchased in 1997 and used to create the Fort Corchaug and Downs Farm Preserve (631-734-6413). Visitors can explore the area and experience a bit of the culture of its original inhabitants, as well as learn more about its current landowners.

If you're looking to get on the water and see Cutchogue's beauty for yourself, numerous launch sites exist along its shore. The small beach at the end of Main Street, off New Suffolk Avenue in New Suffolk, is a great place to put in if you're headed to Robins Island or Cutchogue's Nassau Point. Follow Little Neck Road or Mason Drive to its end, and you'll find two more spots perfect for getting on the water. My usual put-in whenever I paddle here is at the end of Pequash Avenue, next to Fleet's Neck Beach. While the street parking is limited, the views of Cutchogue Harbor and Robins Island are breathtaking. And if you can tear yourself away from them long enough to launch your kayak, you'll be situated perfectly for a

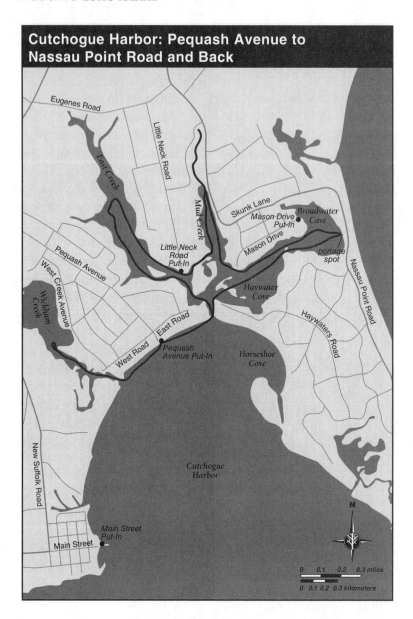

Cutchogue Harbor: Pequash Avenue to Nassau Point Road and Back

trip to Robins Island, around Nassau Point, or along the harbor's shoreline and its side creeks.

USGS Quadrangles
SOUTHOLD (NY)

6 **DESCRIPTION** Launch from the beach at the end of Pequash Avenue, and the first thing you'll have to do is decide on a direction in which to head. The northern tip of Robins Island lies just 2 miles due south of the beach, and the Little Hog Neck peninsula sits on the opposite side of the horseshoe-shaped harbor even closer than that. Then there are four

Pequash Avenue to Nassau Point Road and Back

Level	1A
Distance	6.3 miles round-trip
Time	3 hours
Navigable months	Year-round
Hazards	Boat traffic
Portages	None
Rescue access	Easy
Tidal conditions	Any
Scenery	B+

creeks and coves only 0.5 mile to the northeast, with at least 6 miles of shoreline ready for exploring. All are worthy destinations, but my favorite first stop is the waters of Wickham Creek, just 0.25 mile to the west.

The paddle to Wickham Creek is quick and easy from your put-in. Just follow the developed shoreline to the right (west), and its entrance will appear immediately after two small docks jut out into the harbor. Skirt around them, pass between the rocks to your right, and the sandy beach to the left, and you'll be on Wickham Creek. Unfortunately, the very first thing you'll encounter is a decent-sized marina that takes up a good chunk of the eastern shoreline. It should make you feel better, though, that the opposite shore is completely undeveloped and is perfect for a sea kayak. Its marsh, albeit tiny, holds many nooks and crannies that are just the right size for paddling. Poke around them a bit and you just may be lucky enough to spy a great blue heron, great egret, or any number of shorebirds along the way.

As you paddle deeper into Wickham Creek, the marina quickly fades away. You'll pass a rustic-looking log cabin just after the marina's last dock, followed by a narrowing of land before the creek opens up into a fairly wide body of water that is 0.25 mile wide and almost 0.4 mile long. A glance to the right reveals a shoreline dotted with houses, although they are set back and are far apart enough that they don't distract from the creek's natural feel. It's the land to the left, though, that's quite special. It has been owned by the Wickham family, from whom the creek gets its name, for the past 350 years. In fact, the farm they run there contains some of the oldest continuously cultivated land in the entire United States. The Wickhams are famous for their fruit, which you can buy if you visit their farm by car (more info: 631-734-6441; **wickhamsfruitfarm.com**).

Once you've explored enough of Wickham Creek, retrace your paddle strokes and head back out onto Cutchogue Harbor. Turn your bow to the left (east) and follow the shoreline for 0.5 mile, and you'll come to the other creeks and coves mentioned earlier. Should you be tired and looking for a place to stop and stretch your

GPS COORDINATES

Put-in/take-out
N41° 00.342' W72° 27.897'
Tide station
New Suffolk, NY
N40° 59.502' W72° 28.302'

legs, avoid the private beach on the west side of the inlet, which sports numerous NO TRESPASSING signs. Not to worry—just across the way is another beach that bears no such signs and is the ideal place to take a break.

Stay to the left as you pass through the cove's mouth, and you'll come to a section known as East Creek. It stretches almost 1 mile to the north and is lined almost continuously with waterfront homes, their docks, and their boats, although its southeastern corner supports a very small salt marsh. If you find yourself in this marsh, navigate to its opposite side and you'll find the area's other stream, Mud Creek, just to the north. At first glance, Mud Creek will look almost identical to East Creek, bustling with houses and the like. Keep going, though, and you'll soon come to one of Cutchogue's hidden gems.

Few people know that Mud Creek narrows at its northern end to only a few feet and begins winding its way through a secluded, almost wild marsh that is unbelievably beautiful. The area, owned and protected by The Nature Conservancy, boasts wide expanses of spartina grasses and phragmites to the east and dense groves of oak trees to the west, making it the perfect place to view wildlife. The last time I paddled here, I counted almost a dozen great blue herons and great egrets, and I even surprised a white-tailed deer standing on-shore.

Paddle back down Mud Creek and hang a left when you hit the marsh at its beginning to find the piece of water known as Haywater Cove. Its shores are developed, like the two creeks before it, but it does lead to some undeveloped property and another small cove. This final stretch of water, called Broadwater

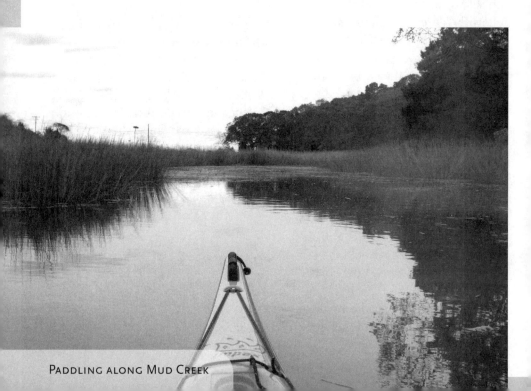

PADDLING ALONG MUD CREEK

Cove, ends at the causeway to Little Hog Neck. Land your kayak there and walk across the causeway to Nassau Point Beach on the other side. The view from its sand is simply stunning. It's also a good place to portage if you're considering circumnavigating the Little Hog Neck peninsula. If not, it's the last stop along your exploration of Cutchogue Harbor, and your turnaround point.

From the beach, the Pequash Avenue put-in is only 1 mile away.

✧ **SHUTTLE DIRECTIONS** To get to the put-in on Cutchogue Harbor, take NY 25 into the village of Cutchogue (3 miles east of Mattituck). Turn right onto Pequash Avenue and follow it to the harbor 1.2 miles later. Park along the side of the road and follow the small trail down to the beach.

7 FLANDERS BAY

✧ **OVERVIEW** Almost entirely within Suffolk County parkland, the southern shore of Flanders Bay makes up one of the largest undeveloped wetland ecosystems on all of Long Island. It stretches almost 3 miles as the crow flies, although an amazing 8 miles of shoreline is packed in that same area along the four major creeks—Goose, Birch, Mill, and Hubbard—that meander through Hubbard County Park's vast marsh system. Together, the bay's shores, its creeks' banks, its salt marsh, and its woodlands of cedar, pine, maple, and oak create an incredibly diverse area that is one of the most valuable fish and wildlife habitats throughout the entire Peconic Bay system.

It was this diversity of life that first attracted settlers to the park site 10,000 years ago and still attracts visitors today. Thankfully, the creation of Hubbard County Park has preserved this ecologically important area and ensured that it will remain a Long Island treasure to be enjoyed for generations to come. Hikers, bird-watchers, nature photographers, and fishermen alike have long taken advantage of the park and its access to Flanders Bay. More recently, it has become quite a popular destination for the paddling crowd.

Flanders Bay contains a significant amount of unprotected water, which can get a bit choppy whenever the wind picks up. Nevertheless, its creeks are almost always calm and serene during most conditions and can provide paddlers with great places to kayak on those days when paddling on open water is not an option. You can launch from any of three excellent put-ins: at the end of Pine Avenue, at the end of Birch Creek Road, or off Red Creek Road. All are free and open to everyone.

USGS Quadrangles
MATTITUCK (NY)

7 **DESCRIPTION** It's hard to imagine just how pristine the area before you is when you stand near the put-in at the end of Pine Avenue, especially

Pine Avenue to
Red Creek Park and Back

Level	2B
Distance	10.1 miles round-trip
Time	4 hours
Navigable months	Year-round
Hazards	Open water, boat traffic
Portages	None
Rescue access	Limited
Tidal conditions	4 hours before or after high tide
Scenery	A+

considering the multitude of houses that sit behind you. Hit the water and head around Goose Creek Point, though, and you'll soon be immersed in the bay's natural beauty. Then, if you stay tight along the sandy shore of the point, paddling past the mosquito ditches dug through the salt marsh that borders the land, you'll enter one of Flanders' finest paddling spots, Birch Creek, just 0.4 mile later.

As you paddle Birch Creek, you'll notice that it seems to be more of a cove than a creek at first. Still only a few hundred feet across at this point, the creek does stay open a bit before it funnels down into a much narrower stretch, but not before passing more of the sprawling salt marsh that dominates the area. Keep looking to your right (south) as you paddle through this highly productive zone, and you should spy a small beach connected to Birch Creek Road, a dirt path that leads south. Birch Creek Road connects

NY 24 to the beach, making it an excellent put-in. In fact, it is often used by paddlers wanting to explore the creek and the waters beyond.

Use the beach as a rest stop or to adjust any gear before paddling farther. Then paddle past the sand and into the narrower part of Birch Creek to enter what seems like a completely different world. The spartina of the outer marsh remains, although it is less widespread here than on the outer portion of the creek. As you gaze past the marsh, you'll also notice that it's closely bordered by a dense grove of trees. Oaks predominate on the creek's western side, whereas the eastern side is lined mostly with pitch pines. Follow this slender stretch of water and enjoy its views for almost 0.4 mile. It then dead-ends just before NY 24—which is for the best anyway, considering everything else Flanders Bay has in store for you.

To reach the next stream, known as Mill Creek, you'll have to retrace your paddle strokes and enter Flanders Bay once again. Look to your right just before you do so, and you should see a small cluster of trees beyond the widespread salt marsh mentioned earlier. Those trees roughly mark Mill Creek's entrance, although you'll have to paddle around the ragged piece of

GPS Coordinates

Put-in/take-out
N40° 54.315' W72° 35.516'
Tide station
Shinnecock Canal, NY
N40° 54.000' W72° 30.000'

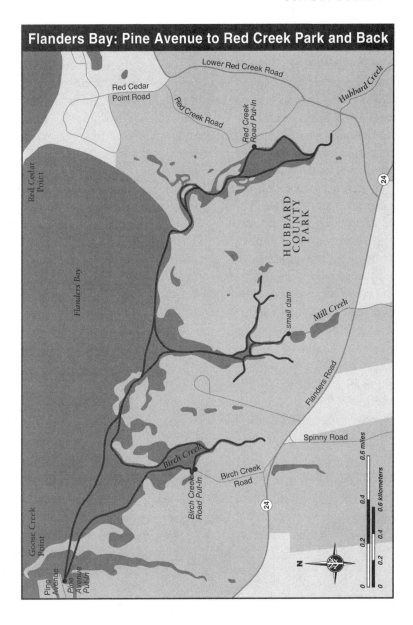

Flanders Bay: Pine Avenue to Red Creek Park and Back

Lower Red Creek Road

Red Cedar Point Road

Red Creek Road

Red Creek Road Put-In

Hubbard Creek

Red Cedar Point

24

HUBBARD COUNTY PARK

Flanders Bay

small dam

Mill Creek

Flanders Road

Spinny Road

0.6 miles

0.6 kilometers

0.4

0.4

0.2

0.2

0

0

Birch Creek

Birch Creek Road Put-In

Birch Creek Road

24

Goose Creek Point

Pine Avenue

Pine Avenue Put-In

N

land that supports these trees to gain access to it. Take care when rounding the point, as some sandy shoals sit just beneath the water's surface, ready to stop your momentum and put a scratch or two in your boat.

A small cluster of cabins comes in to view as you round the point and begin paddling due south into Mill Creek, though you shouldn't be discouraged by this intrusion. Although they were once used by members of a private hunting and fishing club, the buildings are now used to house biologists and conservation workers, whose goals include preserving and protecting the very area you're paddling through. Head past the cabins and farther into the creek, and you'll notice that it branches off in four separate directions. Option one, to the right (west), leads just a short distance into the heart of a thick spartina marsh before it becomes impassable. Option two, to the southwest, similarly dead-ends rather quickly at a fairly tall wall of phragmites. The other two options are quite interesting, though, and enjoyable to paddle.

Head down the branch at the creek's southeastern corner, and you'll be able to paddle for 0.2 mile, winding your way along a narrow passageway that ultimately leads to an old dam holding back the water from a small but pretty phragmites-lined pond beyond. Soak up the scenery as much as you want, then back out and head down the last of the branches, where the landscape only gets prettier. Twist

and turn your way 0.2 mile down the stream, and you'll come to a fork. Head south here and you'll soon find your bow encountering an impenetrable wall of vegetation, obliging you to back-paddle until you have enough room to turn completely around. Head north at the fork, though, and you'll get another 0.2 mile of water to paddle before reaching a stunning little pond ringed with phragmites and likely hiding a huge group of black ducks. Then paddle back to Flanders Bay once more, following the narrow sliver of sand on your right (east) to Hubbard Creek, the last of the area's creeks.

Unlike the entrances to Mill Creek and Birch Creek, the entrance to Hubbard Creek is quite narrow, with a fairly significant tidal current that may either help or hinder your forward momentum depending on which way it's flowing. Once you've made it through, an interesting mix of

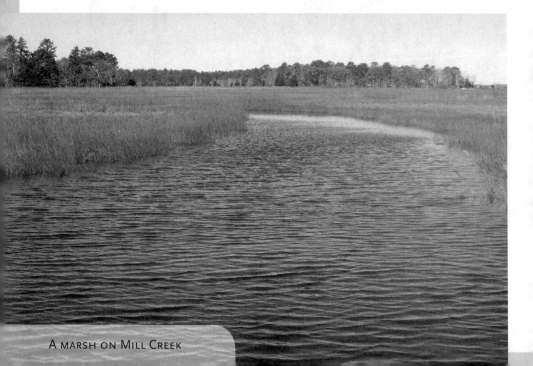

A MARSH ON MILL CREEK

mosquito ditches, grass islands, and winding channels stretches out before you and presents a multitude of nooks and crannies to explore. This maze of a marsh is relegated mostly to the creek's northern half, becoming more uniform the farther south you paddle, though the whole of the creek is bordered by thickly growing oaks and pitch pines and lined with tall phragmites reeds.

A small dock sits a few dozen paddle strokes down the creek's eastern shore, a bit north of a tiny path that leads to the water's edge from nearby Red Creek Road. This is the water access you'll use should you choose to launch your boat from Hubbard County Park instead of off Pine Avenue the next time you paddle here. Paddle past this path now and head toward the creek's southwest corner, where it reaches its narrowest point. This shallow, tightly coiled stretch of creek is truly the perfect place to observe a classic Pine Barrens forest, with pitch pines and oaks growing in abundance right down to the water's edge.

Unfortunately, this portion of Hubbard Creek becomes impassable at Red Creek Road, bringing your trip south to an end. It also marks the last section of water along this stretch of Flanders Bay, and the ultimate turnaround point of your paddle. You must head back to Flanders Bay one final time, then point your bow west and paddle the 1.7 miles back to Pine Avenue and your car.

✧ **SHUTTLE DIRECTIONS** To get to the put-in on Flanders Bay, take I-495 (the Long Island Expressway) to Exit 72 (Riverhead). Follow the exit ramp to NY 25 and head east 3.4 miles into Riverhead. Turn right onto NY 24 and follow it to a traffic circle 0.1 mile later. Go around the circle and continue east on NY 24, the fifth road off the circle. Turn left onto Longneck Boulevard after 3.3 miles, and follow it north for 0.6 mile before turning right onto Pine Avenue. Take Pine Avenue to its end at the water's edge, and park anywhere along the shoulder.

8 FORGE RIVER

✧ **OVERVIEW** The Forge is a short but wide river on Long Island's South Shore, near the village of Mastic. Created about 20,000 years ago when Long Island was being carved out by glaciers, it now flows about 3 miles before it empties into the tidal lagoon known as Moriches Bay, protected from the ravages of the Atlantic Ocean by Long Island's barrier beaches. When an opening in that barrier was created by a storm in 1931, forming what is now Moriches Inlet, an influx of ocean water allowed the Forge to take on new life as a saltwater estuary, acted on by the tides twice a day.

Since its formation, the Forge has been a shallow river. Throughout its history, it has rarely exceeded more than a few feet deep, and it seems to have only gotten shallower with time. The damming of the river near its northern end to create West Mill

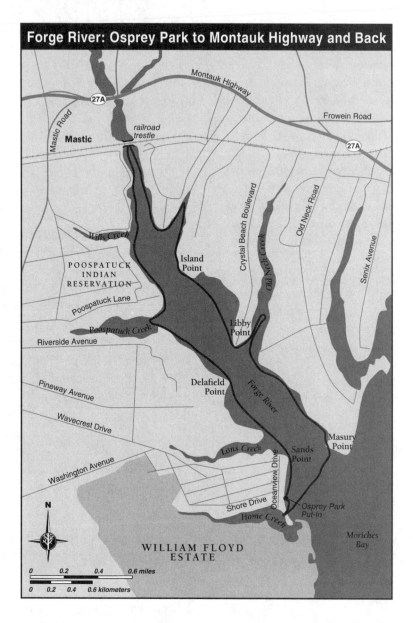

Forge River: Osprey Park to Montauk Highway and Back

Pond is believed to have started a gradual filling-in of the Forge, greatly slowing down the river's already sluggish flow and allowing silt to build up. Over time, the ends of the river's side creeks began to fill in as well, severely limiting the water exchange that could take place and fostering stagnation.

Unfortunately, conditions on the Forge River only got worse from there. Many people began to settle along its protected shores, bringing with them all of the problems associated with human development. Then duck farming began to flourish on neighboring lands, adding even more fertilizers, organic wastes, and other pollutants to the river. With little water flow to flush any contaminants away, the river began to accumulate these toxins in dangerous amounts. The opening of Moriches Inlet did improve the water flow somewhat, and dredging portions of the river has helped as well; nevertheless, the Forge is still feeling the effects of its environmental problems.

Recently, the rallying cry "Save the Forge River!" has been used to marshal help and support in restoring and protecting the waterway. The conservation group that coined that slogan, Save the Forge River, Inc., is fighting for the river's well-being. Increased flow, a storm-water management plan, improvements in septic systems, and wetland rehabilitation are just a few of the organization's goals. Its members have their work cut out for them, but their cause is not a lost one.

Thankfully, the Forge still has a lot to offer. Beautiful, albeit small, sections of salt marsh dot its shores. A good number of finfish still call the river's waters home, and herons, egrets, terns, and gulls are still frequently encountered along its banks. There are even populations of ospreys and bitterns that nest along the river. Boaters enjoy cruising some of its waters, swimmers dive under its waves, and fishermen have returned to its beaches.

Should you want to experience the Forge for yourself, there is no better put-in than Osprey Park in the town of Brookhaven. Near the mouth of the river, the park has bathroom facilities, a large fishing pier, a small beach, and enough parking to accommodate a flotilla of kayakers.

Osprey Park to Montauk Highway and Back

Level	1B
Distance	6.4 miles round-trip
Time	3 hours
Navigable months	Year-round
Hazards	Boat traffic
Portages	None
Rescue access	Easy
Tidal conditions	Any
Scenery	C

USGS Quadrangles
MORICHES (NY)

8 **DESCRIPTION** As you look out from the beach at Osprey Park, the development that is so prevalent along the Forge River is quite hard to miss. There are houses almost everywhere you look, except for a small section of wooded shoreline directly across from the park, and the land of the William Floyd Estate just to the south.

Built in 1718, the 613-acre estate was first a plantation. Later it became the private hunting and fishing preserve of the Floyd family and has remained in the family for more than 300 years. Thankfully, the Floyds did little to alter the land, especially near

GPS COORDINATES

Put-in/take-out
N40° 46.409' W72° 48.852'
Tide station
Moriches Inlet, NY
N40° 45.900' W72° 45.198'

the river, leaving its forest, fields, and salt marsh mainly intact. Head south immediately upon launching from Osprey Park and you'll be able to witness the natural beauty of the Floyd Estate firsthand.

A natural transition between old and new, the creek just south of Osprey Park, known as Home Creek, contains a somewhat developed northern shore, with houses, docks, and a small marina lining the way. On the other hand, the opposite shore, bordering the Floyd Estate, is completely natural, with a thin line of spartina grass separating the water from a dense woodland. It's too bad that Home Creek runs for only about 0.75 mile before it ends, as it's quite a stunning bit of water to paddle. The land beyond is just as enjoyable to explore by kayak, although it's more marsh than forest. This area is about

twice as long as Home Creek and can easily add a few miles to your trip should you want to venture farther into Moriches Bay. But if venturing upstream on the Forge River is your goal, turn around and close the 0.5-mile gap between where you are and the river's eastern bank.

A few houses line this stretch of river, although they're a bit bigger and more obscured than most of the others you'll see. Look back far enough through the heavy hedge and grass cover, and you should be able to make some of them out. At the very least, you'll be able to see their docks, which you'll have to paddle around. Still, the river maintains a somewhat natural feel along this stretch, with some spartina grasses growing along the sandy shore before a sparse stand of cherry, birch, and cedar trees. Most

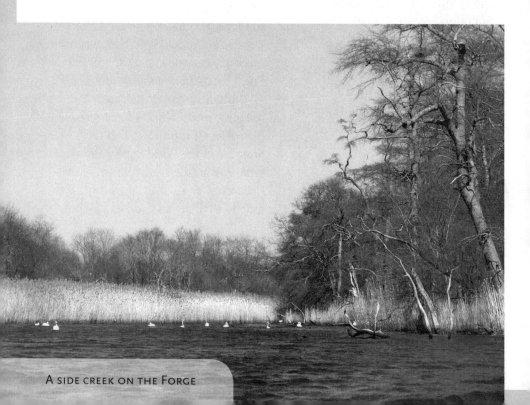

A SIDE CREEK ON THE FORGE

of that changes 0.5 mile beyond the river's mouth, where the mostly green shoreline is replaced by man-made bulkheads designed to protect the tightly packed houses built right on the water's edge.

These dozen or so homes lead the way to the first side creek along the Forge's eastern side. Called Old Neck Creek, it runs almost 1 mile to the north before ending at a wall of vegetation. Paddle it and you'll first encounter a large marina at its beginning, followed by scores of homes along both sides. Throw in the docks that are associated with almost every house, and this side creek will suddenly feel very crowded.

Thankfully, the next side creek along the Forge, just 0.5 mile farther north, is much prettier. Whereas I encountered only lawnmowers and loud music when I last paddled Old Neck Creek, I chanced upon a gorgeous great blue heron and a large group of black ducks hiding out along a secluded stretch of this second creek. Unfortunately, it is only long enough to allow about 0.5 mile of paddling.

Once you come out of this second creek, there is only 0.6 mile of developed river left before you reach a railroad trestle. A small pond ringed with phragmites sits on the trestle's northern side, pretty enough to warrant at least a cursory examination. It is also the northernmost limit of the Forge River, and thus the turnaround point of the paddle.

You'll likely find your trip south along the river's western shore very similar to your paddle up its eastern shore. Small houses line almost every

inch of available space along the water, with their bulkheads, docks, and boats jutting out onto the river itself. Even the next creek just south of the Forge River Boat Club, known as Wills Creek, does little to break the monotony, as it also contains much of the same scenery. Not until 0.5 mile later does something new and interesting appear: the Poospatuck Indian Reservation.

On the north shore of Poospatuck Creek, the reservation, or what little you will be able to see of it, is the smallest Indian reservation in New York State. It consists of about 70 acres of land, with a large dock and a few buildings visible from the water. Although there is little in the way of traditional Native American culture to be seen, paddling beside such a reservation is a unique experience.

Once you pass the reservation, the houses on the Forge seem to grow in size and back away from the water once again. Thus, the riverbanks take on a more natural feel for the last mile of paddling before you return to Osprey Park.

◇ **SHUTTLE DIRECTIONS** To get to the put-in in Osprey Park, take NY 27 (Sunrise Highway) to Exit 58S (CR 46/William Floyd Parkway). Take the William Floyd Parkway south 0.2 mile and turn left onto NY 27A (Montauk Highway). Continue east on NY 27A for 1.6 miles before turning right onto Mastic Road. Follow Mastic Road south 1.8 miles and turn left onto Wavecrest Drive. Continue on Wavecrest until it ends after 1.8 miles, and turn right onto Oceanview Drive. Osprey Park is at the end of Oceanview Drive.

9 GEORGICA POND

◇ **OVERVIEW** Georgica Pond may be one of the most unusual bodies of water on Long Island. On the south shore of East Hampton town, the 290-acre pond is actually a lagoon, separated from the Atlantic Ocean only by a narrow strip of barrier beach. What makes the pond unique, though, is the unstable nature of its separation from the ocean. Quite often breaks form in the beach, opening Georgica Pond to an influx of salt water from the Atlantic. Sometimes the result of natural occurrences and other times due to man's actions, the openings rapidly change the chemistry of the water and create an environment more estuary-like than pondlike. These conditions remain throughout the days or months the pond is connected to the sea, helping create a distinctive plant and animal habitat.

Like most fertile bodies of water on Long Island, Georgica Pond had a group of Native Americans—the Shinnecocks, in this case—inhabiting its environs. (The pond gets its name from one member of the tribe, a man named Jeorgkee, who lived along its shores.) Realizing the bounty of food that could be harvested from the pond's waters and surrounding lands, Europeans eventually purchased the Shinnecocks' territory and began fishing and farming it.

As time wore on, the town of East Hampton, including the land around Georgica Pond, became more and more populated, and developments began to pop up everywhere. The area became a haven for the rich and famous along the way, earning the "Hamptons" distinction that we know today. Amazingly, though, the waterfront of Georgica Pond has retained much of its original appeal. Sure, wealthy people and celebrities have built sprawling homes along its shores, but because most did so to find respite from the spotlight, they've worked to keep the setting serene and relatively unspoiled. There are no docks on the pond, nor are there powerboats of any sort. Not even a single road is visible from its waters. In short, Georgica Pond is a sanctuary in the midst of the East End craziness.

Paddling here has become quite popular in recent years. A convenient put-in is right off Montauk Highway, where a small creek flows alongside a roadside turnoff and empties into the pond. The water is accessible most times of the year and can make for a great way to spend a day during any season. Just be sure to bring your family, a picnic, and a bathing suit.

USGS Quadrangles
EAST HAMPTON (NY)

9 DESCRIPTION Although Georgica Pond proper is an interesting paddle, its two coves and four creeks are the truly exciting parts to explore. Launching from the small lot on Montauk Highway puts you immediately on one of those creeks: 0.25-mile-long Tallmage's Creek. Unfortunately, it can get quite shallow when water levels

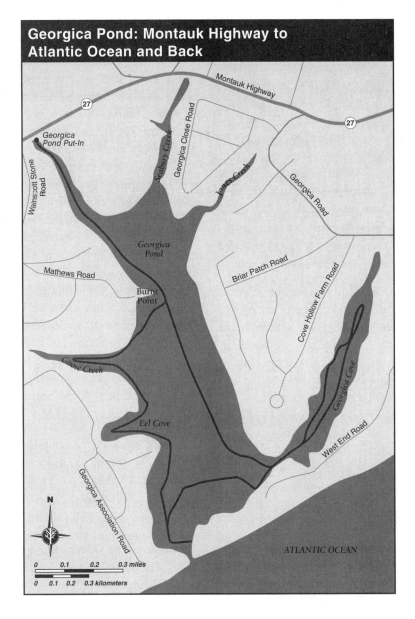

Georgica Pond: Montauk Highway to Atlantic Ocean and Back

Montauk Highway

27

27

Georgica Close Road

Sydney Creek

James Creek

Georgica Pond Put-In

Wainscott Stone Road

Georgica Road

Georgica Pond

Mathews Road

Briar Patch Road

Burnt Point

Cove Hollow Farm Road

Goose Creek

Georgica Cove

Eel Cove

West End Road

Georgica Association Road

N

ATLANTIC OCEAN

0   0.1   0.2   0.3 miles

0   0.1   0.2   0.3 kilometers

---

are low, and you may have to walk your boat a few hundred feet to deeper waters. Don't despair, though. Instead, take the time to enjoy the beautiful oak, maple, and willow trees that line the creek's western shore. Pay close attention to the eastern shore as well: the artist who owns the property has decorated it with assorted sculptures and large pieces of art. It's not every day that a paddler can enjoy both nature and culture from the seat of a kayak.

As Tallmage's Creek makes its way toward the main pond, look to the trees on the right to catch glimpses of the various shorebirds that call Georgica Pond home. On my last

Montauk Highway to Atlantic Ocean and Back

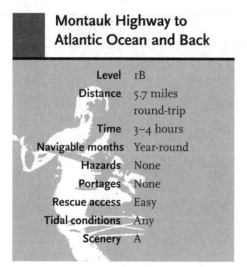

Level	1B
Distance	5.7 miles round-trip
Time	3–4 hours
Navigable months	Year-round
Hazards	None
Portages	None
Rescue access	Easy
Tidal conditions	Any
Scenery	A

midsummer paddle here, I counted at least a dozen great egrets sitting among the trees' branches, their crisp white feathers easily giving away their location. I also saw a few great blue herons, as well as two ospreys.

Although swans are somewhat commonplace on Long Island's waters, those on this section of Georgica Pond warrant special mention. I have heard of more than a few people being attacked by one of the swans that live on the northern pond. Although I've never been attacked myself, nor have I witnessed an attack during the many times I've paddled here, I do feel it is my duty to warn fellow kayakers about these swans. Paddle far away from them, do not feed or engage them in any way, and please refrain from making ugly-duckling jokes within their earshot.

Just south of where Tallmage's Creek opens to the pond, a small spit of land sticks out on the western shore. Known as Burnt Point, it's all that remains of an earthen causeway built by locals to allow easier passage to the pond's opposite shore. The rest of the causeway has

long since eroded, although a small portion sits just a few inches below the water's surface and reaches about midway across. Incidentally, the sprawling home on Burnt Point is one of the most expensive houses in the United States, selling for $45 million. Imagine how many composite kayaks that could buy!

Continue south along the shore and you'll encounter another stream, Goose Creek, 0.4 mile after Burnt Point. It's lined with homes (of a more modest price) tucked among large oak and pine trees that give it a charming, woodsy feel. Swallows and kingfishers abound along this stretch of water. Another of Georgica Pond's branches, Eel Cove, is just 0.25 mile south of Goose Creek. Like the creek, Eel Cove is bordered by small homes, although some of their owners kept gorgeous wooden sail-boats floating just off their properties when I last explored its shores.

After paddling through Eel Cove, look for a feature unique to the pond about 0.5 mile to the south. Georgica Pond periodically opens to the Atlantic Ocean when a break forms in the dunes between them. If such a break is open when you happen to be here, it can mean a good deal of fun. Paddling out to the ocean or surfing the current back in to the pond is always a blast. Regardless of an opening, the beach here is always a fine place to land, take

GPS COORDINATES

Put-in/take-out
N40° 56.989' W72° 14.353'
Tide station
Shinnecock Inlet, NY
N40° 50.298' W72° 28.500'

a rest, and have a bite to eat before continuing up the pond's eastern shore. But don't bypass the next cove, called Georgica Cove, especially if you want to paddle among more of the rich and famous.

The cove branches off the southeasternmost corner of the pond, stretching for more than 0.5 mile to the northeast. It passes more than a dozen beautiful homes along the way, some owned, or previously owned, by celebrities such as Steven Spielberg, Martha Stewart, and Calvin Klein. Even Bill and Hillary Clinton vacationed here during his presidency. I like to try to match the celebrities' personalities with the styles of the houses in an effort to guess where each person lives. Of course, seeing one of them standing on his or her dock waving hello would help too.

From Georgica Cove it's roughly 1 mile to the next two creeks, Jones and Seabury, both in the northeast corner of the pond. The creeks are each about 0.25 mile long and, save for a large house or two, have undisturbed shorelines. Paddle them to their upper reaches, then exit to the pond once again, where the put-in up Tallmage's Creek sits only 0.5 mile distant.

✧ **SHUTTLE DIRECTIONS** The put-in for Georgica Pond is on NY 27 (Montauk Highway), 3.3 miles east of Bridgehampton and 2.6 miles west of East Hampton. Look for the small parking area and creek just east of Wainscott Stone Road.

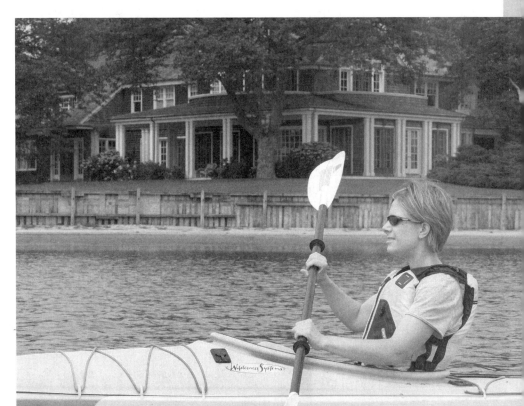

PADDLING PAST ONE OF THE MOST EXPENSIVE HOUSES IN AMERICA

10   GREENPORT HARBOR

✧ **OVERVIEW** The village of Greenport sits on Long Island's North Fork, midway between Southold and Orient, its downtown nestled comfortably on the water's edge and its connection to the sea long and storied. Originally known as Winter Harbor, Greenport was the home port of trade ships traveling to South America before and during the Revolutionary War. It was also an important port for the whaling trade, maintaining a fleet of 24 whalers over a 60-year period. Shipbuilding also helped define the village during the 1800s. But it was the fishing industry that had the most lasting impact on Greenport— fishing boats, processing plants, and oyster shacks were once so numerous here that most of the village retained a perpetual smell of fish.

Thankfully, that unpleasant odor is a thing of the past, although the town's nautical history is still very much alive and ever-present. Travel down Main Street and you'll pass dozens of historic homes that once belonged to ships' captains and their families before you come to the many charming stores and shops that lead to the village's wharf. On this wharf sit a nautical-supply store that has changed little since opening more than 100 years ago, a stunning collection of sailing ships from a bygone era, a small assortment of seafood restaurants, and a waterfront park for all to enjoy.

Of course, with a bustling downtown that caters to tourists, Greenport can be quite crowded during the summer. Its waters can become even busier, with hundreds of boats coming and going in every direction throughout the day. As such, Greenport is a paddling destination best left for fall or spring, when the crowds have gone and most of the boats have moved on. There is still a great deal to see and enjoy during these months, and you'll be better able to relax and take it all in.

Surprisingly, this busy but small seaport provides little in the way of water access for kayakers. The best, and possibly only, put-in is just west of Greenport near its train station. In fact, you'll have to park in the station lot and carry your boat and gear over its low concrete bulkhead to reach the water. But the extra legwork lets you enter the water right at the harbor's edge, primed for a sightseeing paddle along its length or even across to its other side, where Shelter Island's Dering Harbor awaits.

USGS Quadrangles
GREENPORT (NY)

10 **DESCRIPTION** Because Greenport is a very active, working harbor throughout the year, you should take a great deal of caution and care when

GPS COORDINATES

Put-in/take-out
N41° 05.967' W72° 21.751'
Tide station
Greenport, NY
N41° 06.102' W72° 21.702'

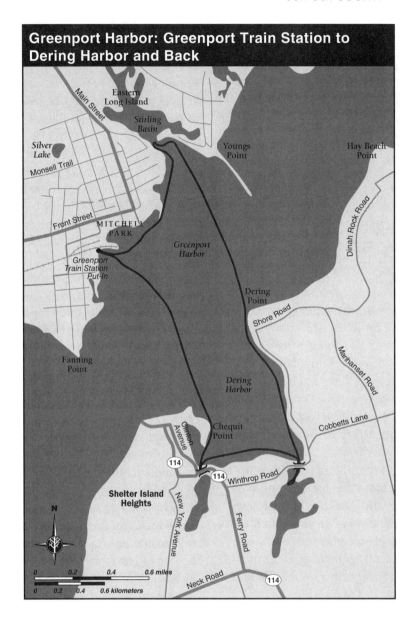

Greenport Harbor: Greenport Train Station to Dering Harbor and Back

Main Street

Eastern
Long Island

Stirling
Basin

Silver
Lake

Monsell Trail

Front Street

MITCHELL
PARK

Greenport
Train Station
Put-In

Fanning
Point

Youngs
Point

Greenport
Harbor

Dering
Point

Shore Road

Dering
Harbor

Clifton
Avenue

Chequit
Point

114

114   Winthrop Road

Shelter Island
Heights

New York Avenue

Ferry Road

Neck Road

114

Cobbetts Lane

Manhanset Road

Dinah Rock Road

Hay Beach
Point

N

0   0.2   0.4   0.6 miles

0   0.2   0.4   0.6 kilometers

launching from the train-station beach, even during the off-season. You'll notice a few fishing trawlers sitting at their docks almost straight ahead, with the Shelter Island North Ferry cruising back and forth just a few feet beyond. Both will have to be paddled past if you're to reach the main docks of Greenport. Assuming you're here during the off-season and there are few other boats to contend with, you'll just have to watch and wait for an opening in the traffic, paddling deliberately and steadily when the way is clear. Once you've left the trawlers and ferry behind, head almost due east

Train Station to Dering Harbor and Back

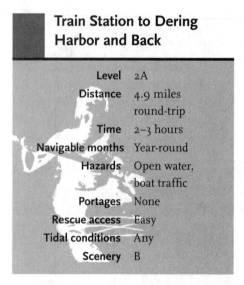

Level	2A
Distance	4.9 miles round-trip
Time	2–3 hours
Navigable months	Year-round
Hazards	Open water, boat traffic
Portages	None
Rescue access	Easy
Tidal conditions	Any
Scenery	B

toward the tip of the long town pier, and you'll be able to slow down and enjoy yourself as soon as you reach it.

Look to your left just before you reach the pier, and you should catch a glimpse of Greenport Village's Mitchell Park. In addition to a marina and boardwalk, this park boasts a beautiful antique carousel and an amazing camera obscura. Both of these amazing structures are open during the summer, and you should definitely check them out after your trip if time permits. Paddle past the park and you'll quickly come to another pier, home to the locally famous Claudio's Clam Bar. In the summer its dock is always crammed with boats, while dozens more wait out in the harbor for a chance to tie up and eat. When Claudio's shuts down in the late fall, its empty pier yields great views of Greenport from the water. The town's rusty side lies just a few hundred feet away, on the other side of another dock where stands a stunning tribute to one of Long Island's most iconic

birds: the osprey. This large sculpture sits atop a small collection of steel beams taken from the World Trade Center's twin towers after they collapsed, making it a somber memorial as well as a notable landmark.

More of Greenport's maritime history comes into view as you paddle around the osprey sculpture and head north toward Greenport's Stirling Basin. The Greenport Yacht and Shipbuilding Company maintains a small boatyard in the village's southeastern corner, storing a handful of modern boats amid quite a few old and derelict vessels. Even the boatyard's buildings seem to be in a state of disrepair, as if exposed to the elements for way too long. Of course, no tetanus shots will be necessary as long as you don't paddle too close to any of the heeling or sunken vessels. Take a few photos, enjoy the glimpse into Greenport's past, and then continue north for a quick trip back to modern times.

Paddle just 0.2 mile farther and you'll be floating just offshore of some fairly new waterfront condos and a small dock. Continue another 0.1 mile farther and you'll pass through the narrow entrance to Greenport's Stirling Basin. Once you've entered the basin, a quick glance around will show you that it is predominantly a large mooring field, lined with docks and marinas almost as far as the eye can see. Some good-looking boats call this body of water home, and boat-lovers will surely enjoy exploring its every nook and cranny. Others may grow bored with Stirling Basin's monotony and seek another source of enjoyment. For them, a paddle across the harbor to Shelter Island's Dering Harbor may be an excellent alternative.

Just a 1-mile paddle due south from Greenport, Dering Harbor seems like a different world. Lined almost entirely with houses and yards instead of large piers, businesses, and restaurants, it has a much more relaxed feel than Greenport's hustle and bustle. With the harbor's more than 1.5 miles of shoreline to explore, a quaint little business district tucked away into one corner, and two decent-sized ponds accessible by paddling under two separate bridges, spending a lot of time here is quite an easy thing to do.

Once you've finished exploring all that Dering Harbor has to offer, it'll be time to head back to Greenport Harbor. The crossing from Dering's westernmost tip, Chequit Point, to Greenport's train station is only 1 mile long, although it does require you to cross the Shelter Island North Ferry's path once more. Once again, let the ferry pass well in front of you and then continue north, back to the train station beach and your take-out.

✧ **SHUTTLE DIRECTIONS** To get to your put-in at Greenport's train station, pick up NY 25 at its intersection with the village's Main Street and travel 0.25 mile west. Turn left onto Fourth Street, cross the tracks, and turn left again into the station's lot. Park as close as you can to the water, and carry your boat and gear over the low concrete wall at the water's edge.

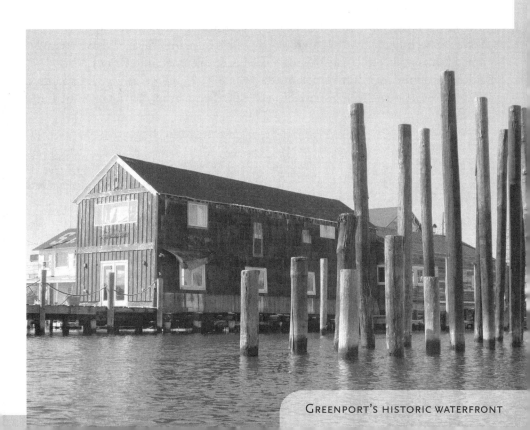

GREENPORT'S HISTORIC WATERFRONT

11 HALLOCK BAY

✧ **OVERVIEW** Throughout history, many people have described Long Island as fish-shaped, with the head of the fish facing to the west and tail to the east. Orient Point, then, represents the tip of the upper tail fin—as far east as one can go on the island's North Fork. Indeed, nothing but a few islands lies beyond this point, about 100 miles east of New York City. Sure, many refer to Long Island's other point, Montauk, as "The End." But though it's not as far east as Montauk, Orient is still quite a drive from most places and might deserve a label of its own.

So what can you expect to find after driving all of the way out to the North Fork's easternmost town? Numerous small farmstands punctuate the roadsides. An abundance of historic homes fills the countryside. And a sense of attachment to the many nearby bodies of water permeates the area. In fact, even though Orient was originally named *Poquatuck* after the tribe who lived there, its name was later changed by the Europeans to Oysterponds out of respect to the water and its predominant species.

Its name was changed once more to the current Orient, but the village has never lost its close ties to the water. Scores of fishing boats call Orient home, plying its bays and harbors for the many species that live there. Shellfishing is as popular now as it always was. A ferry service runs trips to Connecticut and other New England destinations. And a gorgeous state park showcases Orient's pristine beachfront. It truly is a maritime playground.

Although once banned as a preventative measure, kayakers have recently been welcomed into Orient Beach State Park and can access the waters of Orient Harbor, Gardiners Bay, and

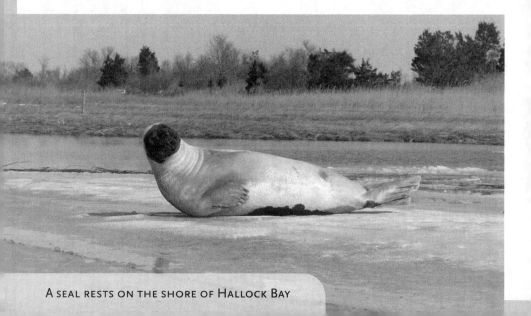

A SEAL RESTS ON THE SHORE OF HALLOCK BAY

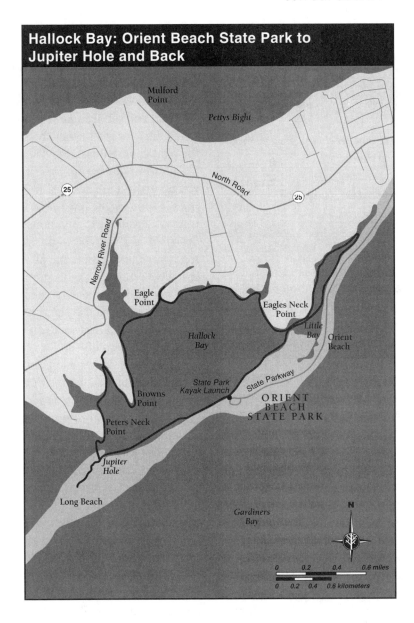

Hallock Bay: Orient Beach State Park to Jupiter Hole and Back

Hallock Bay from its 2.5-mile-long beachfront. Along with its bathroom facilities, picnic areas, playgrounds, and walking paths, the park has also added a designated kayak launch site that rents boats to interested paddlers. This put-in sits on the Hallock Bay side of the park, providing easy access to its calm and protected waters and its salt marshes and cedar groves. It is also the ideal spot for anyone wanting to paddle to the nearby Long Beach Bar Lighthouse, or "Bug Light," as it is affectionately known.

USGS Quadrangles
ORIENT (NY), GREENPORT (NY)

Orient State Park to Jupiter Hole and Back

Level	1B
Distance	7 miles round-trip
Time	3 hours
Navigable months	Year-round
Hazards	None
Portages	None
Rescue access	Limited
Tidal conditions	Any
Scenery	A+

11 DESCRIPTION Although the Orient Beach State Park kayak launch is actually just a small trail leading down the beach to the water, it is well situated almost midway, east to west, along Hallock Bay's southern shore. Thus, you may choose to head in either direction upon launching your kayak from its beach: east toward the bay's deepest reaches or west toward its mouth. Although you can travel in only one direction, there's no need to worry about missing out on a portion of the bay. Because of its small size, you can easily paddle around the bay's perimeter and enjoy its every nook and cranny.

If you choose to go west along the bay's Long Beach peninsula first, you'll be paddling along an incredibly pristine and beautiful shore. Nothing but the gentle sound of waves lapping against the pebbly beach will fill your ears while nothing but an uninterrupted wilderness will lie before you. In fact, there is not a single sign of civilization along the remainder of the peninsula, save for a sign or two posted along the tree line. Instead, little more than sand, spartina grass, and cedar trees stretches for 2.5 miles to the tip of land at Long Beach Point. Follow this gorgeous stretch of waterfront, and you'll soon be poised to make the short (0.1-mile) crossing to the iconic Long Beach Bar Lighthouse.

Interestingly, the light you'll see if you do make it to Long Beach Point is not the same as the one that was built in 1871. This original lighthouse was designed as a screwpile light, meaning it was built upon metal pilings that were screwed into the ground as supports. Imagine what the light would have looked like standing atop numerous piling legs—like an insect skimming the water—and it's easy to see how it earned its nickname, "Bug Light." The concrete foundation that the light sits upon now was added years later as an improvement to the structure. Unfortunately, the original lighthouse was destroyed, except for its foundation, in a 1963 fire. The version you see today is a replica, constructed to look exactly the same as its predecessor.

If paddling to Long Beach Point and Bug Light isn't a priority on your trip around Hallock Bay, perhaps exploring Jupiter Hole is on your itinerary. Just east of the bay's narrow mouth on the Long Beach side, the area lies down a small, almost hidden

GPS COORDINATES

Put-in/take-out
N41° 07.813' W72° 16.034'
Tide station
Orient, NY
N41° 08.202' W72° 18.402'

tidal creek that winds its way through a vast section of salt marsh. As you enter the creek, stay to the right when it forks and you'll have a short (0.2-mile) paddle to the salt pond that sits at its end. Along the way, you'll float past a stunning line of red cedar trees that seem to lead the way deeper into this amazing spot. Between the cedar trees, the verdant green marsh, the placid water, and the wildlife you'll likely encounter, Jupiter Hole may be one of the most unforgettable places you'll paddle on Long Island.

After reveling in the beauty of Jupiter Hole or the architecture of the Bug Light, cross the bay's mouth and you'll find a series of small coves that are also quite worthy of your time. The first you'll encounter is shaped much like a U, with two arms that stretch into the marsh to the north. Head for the large grove of oak trees visible to the north, and you'll find yourself at the junction of these two arms, ready to navigate either one. Both arms also contain dozens of mosquito ditches and narrow channels that were cut through the marsh, creating a veritable maze of potential routes. Of course, many do not lead very far, ending quite abruptly in walls of green. Others are navigable for some distance, like the small creek that almost bisects Peters Neck Point or the one that completely separates the oak grove mentioned earlier from the mainland. Either way, it's easy to spend a great deal of time along this small section of Hallock Bay.

If you can tear yourself from this first cove, a second sits just around Browns Point. It stretches more than 0.5 mile north from the bay, bordered on the west by Narrow River Road and on the east by farmland. Unlike its neighbor, this cove has few creeks or channels to explore, but its shoreline is still an attractive place to paddle along.

Continue your clockwise trip around Hallock Bay and you will come to its widest portion just east of Eagle Point. Like Long Beach to the south, this shoreline is remarkably undeveloped, with phragmites and spartina grass growing in a vast marsh surrounded by large stands of oak trees. There are also numerous breaks in the marsh, the biggest being the mouth of a small creek 1 mile east of Eagle Point. If you paddle up this creek, you'll encounter an immense salt marsh on its left side and a low, sandy berm lined with red cedar trees on its right. The berm outlines more farmland, running almost 0.5 mile around the peninsula that almost completely blocks Hallock Bay from Little Bay.

Follow the berm to the south, and eventually to the east, and you will gain access to Little Bay and another 2 miles of navigable shoreline to enjoy. In fact, Little Bay is remarkable enough that it could be a paddling destination in itself. When I last paddled here, on a cold winter day, I saw a common loon and dozens of black and long-tailed ducks, buffleheads, and common mergansers, as well as a pair of red-tailed hawks circling overhead. Most notably, I encountered three harp seals sleeping on large slabs of ice grounded on the Little Bay shore. Unfortunately, the end of Little Bay also marks the last destination of the trip, though 1.5 more miles of paddling remain to get back to the state-park kayak launch.

◇ **SHUTTLE DIRECTIONS** To get to the put-in at Orient Beach State Park, take NY 25 to the village of Orient and continue to Orient Point. Just before the ferry terminal, turn right into the park and follow the road to the westernmost parking lot, where you'll find the kayak-launch site. You'll have to drop your boat and gear off at the launch and park in the lot just a few hundred feet away.

12 HUNTINGTON HARBOR

◇ **OVERVIEW** A longtime favorite of the boating community, Huntington Harbor is yet another body of water on Long Island's North Shore that has become an extremely popular paddling destination as well. Nestled snugly among Oyster Bay, Lloyd Harbor, and Centerport Harbor, it is perfectly situated as the starting point for short family paddles, long day trips, and anything in between.

Although Huntington's original founders likely had no kayaks or paddles in 1653, they definitely knew a good thing when they saw it. They were quick to purchase the land that is now the village of Huntington from the local Matinecock tribe and turn it over to the Europeans already living among the hills, fields, and shoreline. Farming soon began to flourish, a tidal mill was built, and the harbor became a small but bustling seaport. Fast-forward to the 19th century, and the harbor's prominence as a shipbuilding center began to reach its peak. Considering Huntington's proximity to the prosperous whaling port of Cold Spring Harbor, it's no surprise that the town even produced a few whalers of its own.

Adding to Huntington's history and charm is its iconic lighthouse, standing proudly just outside the harbor's entrance. Constructed in 1912, the light was needed to aid the already 55-year-old Lloyd Harbor Light in guiding ships into the harbor's safety. It was built in the Beaux Arts style, looking very much like a castle sitting on the water. With little in the way of modern conveniences or technology, the light was kept running by a hardy lightkeeper for the next 37 years. Unfortunately, its condition deteriorated to the point of being unsafe for occupancy, and the United States Coast Guard considered tearing it down in 1983. Thankfully, the structure was spared an untimely end and is currently undergoing a renovation by the Huntington Lighthouse Preservation Society. This nonprofit group definitely has its work cut out for it and is always looking for volunteers and donations. Look to its website, **huntingtonlight house.org,** for more information or to arrange a tour of this unique structure.

With Huntington having such close ties to the water, one would expect the village to be paddler-friendly, and it is. In fact, it's incredibly easy to launch onto the harbor, either from the town boat ramp or a bit farther north at Goldstar Beach. Although you'll need a municipal parking permit to enter

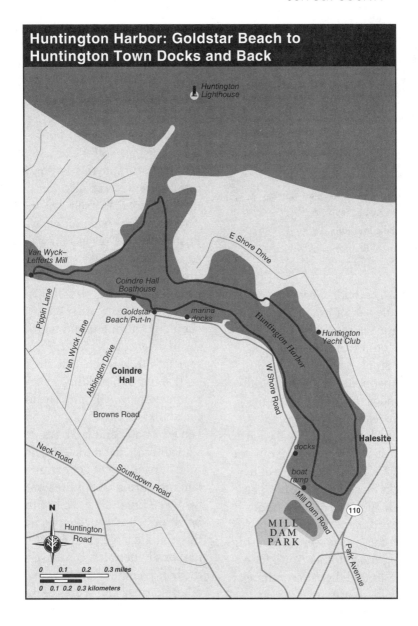

Huntington Harbor: Goldstar Beach to Huntington Town Docks and Back

Huntington Lighthouse

E Shore Drive

Van Wyck–
Lefferts Mill

Coindre Hall Boathouse

Pippin Lane

Goldstar Beach/Put-In

marina docks

Huntington Harbor

Huntington Yacht Club

Van Wyck Lane

Coindre Hall

Abbington Drive

W Shore Road

Browns Road

Halesite

docks

Neck Road

boat ramp

Southdown Road

Mill Dam Road

110

N

Huntington Road

MILL DAM PARK

Park Avenue

0   0.1   0.2   0.3 miles

0   0.1 0.2 0.3 kilometers

Goldstar Beach's lot during the summer, it's open to everyone throughout the rest of the year. The town ramp, on the other hand, is open year-round to one and all. Simply drop your boat and gear off at its side and park anywhere there is room along the side of the road.

USGS Quadrangles
LLOYD HARBOR (NY)

12 **DESCRIPTION** Launching from Goldstar Beach puts you on the water perfectly poised for a paddle west toward the harbor's old mill, north to the harbor's entrance and its

Goldstar Beach to Huntington Town Docks and Back

Level	2A
Distance	4.6 miles round-trip
Time	2 hours
Navigable months	Year-round
Hazards	Boat traffic
Portages	None
Rescue access	Easy
Tidal conditions	Any
Scenery	B

lighthouse beyond, or east into the heart of the harbor itself. Thankfully, Huntington Harbor is small enough (roughly 5 miles of shoreline) that you can simply paddle around the harbor's perimeter and combine all three options into one great trip.

As you leave Goldstar Beach behind and head east along the harbor's southern shore, the first item of interest you'll encounter is a series of five long docks blocking your path. These docks belong to one of the harbor's five major marinas and are usually packed with sailboats and powerboats during the spring and summer. You'll have to paddle around them to continue on your way, so use some care and keep an eye out for moving boats. As always, kayaks have the right of way over any boat with a motor, although I don't know of any paddler who would want to challenge that rule out on the water. Thankfully, the bottleneck as you paddle between the docks and the banks on the opposite shore disappears, and the harbor opens significantly once you've left the marina in your wake.

The harbor also takes a sharp turn to the south just 0.2 mile later. With the incredible number of boats floating on their moorings in this part of the harbor, you'll probably be hugging the shore at this point. There's plenty of room to do so, as the buoys float a decent distance off the beach. Should you desire a route that is a bit more interesting, you can also venture into the mooring field itself and wind your way among the wide variety of boats floating there. This is a no-wake zone, so any moving boat's speed will be limited. Nevertheless, there are always risks inherent with paddling in such close proximity to other boats, and you shouldn't let your attention drift, even if you do encounter a floating party replete with barbecue and drinks.

If you're still paddling close to shore at this point, you'll probably notice the rock bulkhead that lines the boundary between water and land. It's probably a good thing that it took you only 1 mile of paddling to get to this point, as landing during all but the lowest tides would be impossible. Follow the bulkhead south and you'll have a hard time missing the large town docks in the harbor's bottom-left corner. They share the bottom of the harbor with two other marinas and scores of moored boats, as well as the waterfront dining area of the restaurant Prime. Its view

GPS COORDINATES

Put-in/take-out
N40° 53.847' W73° 26.082'
Tide station Lloyd Harbor
Entrance, Huntington Bay, NY
N40° 54.600' W73° 25.902'

is incredible, its food is delicious, and decor is beautiful. Unfortunately, the staff of Prime would surely turn up their noses at anyone settling in for a meal wearing neoprene or GORE-TEX.

Once you pass the restaurant, a few smaller docks are all that remain in the southern portion of Huntington Harbor. So head north again and you'll soon be paddling alongside another unbroken shoreline. Here you can catch a small glimpse of the harbor's history as you glide past the waterfront houses of shipbuilders, captains, and sailors of long ago. You'll spend most of the next 1.5 miles of paddling enjoying the views of these beautiful homes, with only one last set of docks, belonging to the Huntington Yacht Club, in your way.

Look to your right as the shoreline curves north, and you'll have an excellent view of Huntington's busy inlet. You may even see its lighthouse as you begin to paddle across the inlet's mouth. You should also be able to check on the water conditions out on Huntington Bay from here. If there is little to no wind, and thus no whitecaps, a paddle out to the lighthouse may certainly be in order.

If you're skipping the lighthouse, cross the inlet (with great care of course) to gain access to the western portion of the harbor. You'll also have an excellent view of Huntington's Coindre Hall and a good portion of its 34-acre estate. The main building and its sprawling green lawn are both easily visible from the harbor's inlet, but most obvious is the estate's boathouse, perched right on the water's edge. The striking mansion and its boathouse were built in 1912 for George McKesson Brown, a pharmaceutical billionaire, although he lost the property after the stock-market crash of 1929. The estate was then used as a private school before it was taken over by the Suffolk County Department of Parks in 1973. The main hall is in great shape and is often used for grand receptions and weddings. Unfortunately, the boathouse has fallen into disrepair. Boarded windows, graffiti, and broken concrete hide the grandeur of what once was.

Another historic structure sits just 0.5 mile west of Coindre Hall's boathouse, although this one is in much better shape. The barn-shaped Van Wyck–Lefferts Tidal Mill was built by the Van Wyck family in 1795 and has changed little since. It's now owned by The Nature Conservancy, which helps maintain the structure, its original earthen dam, and thankfully, its history. Unless you're participating in one of its guided tours, the conservancy asks that you keep off the mill property and the earthen dam next to it. So take as many pictures as you like, soak in the history, and then simply turn around and head 0.5 mile back to Goldstar Beach and your put-in.

✧ **SHUTTLE DIRECTIONS** To get to the put-in at Goldstar Beach, take the Northern State Parkway to Exit 40N (NY 110). Head north on NY 110 for 5.5 miles until you reach NY 25A. Turn left onto NY 25A and take your first right onto Wall Street. Head north on Wall Street for 0.6 mile, at which point it will turn into West Shore Road.

Continue on West Shore Road for 1.7 miles. The entrance to Goldstar Beach is on the right-hand side of the road.

13 LAKE MONTAUK

⟡ **OVERVIEW** Affectionately known by Long Islanders as "The End," Montauk sits at the tip of the island's South Fork, as far east as one can travel. It is home to an iconic lighthouse commissioned by none other than George Washington, no less than six state parks, the oldest working cattle ranch in the United States, and the largest commercial and sportfishing fleet in New York. Of course, none of these existed hundreds of years ago, when the Montaukett people inhabited the area. Instead, herds of deer, schools of fish, flocks of ducks, and dense forest were the area's main attractions.

As English settlers began colonizing the East End lands during the 17th century, they worked out an agreement with the Montauketts that allowed both parties to share use of the Montauk Peninsula, although they eventually purchased the land for the low sum of 100 pounds. The settlers then began to raise large herds of cattle there, fish the peninsula's waters, and farm a bit as well. During the late 19th century, the army took interest in the area and established a military base near Montauk Point to house soldiers. Most famously, Teddy Roosevelt and his Rough Riders spent time there after returning from the Spanish-American War.

Little else of interest happened here until the 1920s, when an entrepreneur named Carl Fisher took on Montauk as his latest project. Fisher had recently transformed a buggy swamp named Miami Beach into a prime vacation destination and was hoping to do the same to the East End town. As part of his vision for the "Miami Beach of the North," Fisher built roads, houses, and a glamorous hotel that still stands today as Montauk Manor. To create a port capable of accepting oceanbound vessels, he even blasted an opening into the freshwater Lake Wyandanch and renamed it Lake Montauk. Unfortunately, the real estate market went bust, and Fisher's dream never came to fruition. The development of Montauk was set in motion, however, and fortunately it never stopped.

After a brief ownership by the U.S. Navy during World War II, Lake Montauk and its now-saltwater port became home to an ever-growing fleet of fishing boats. Today, the harbor boasts a large number of fishing records, including the biggest fish ever caught on a rod and reel, while the town itself has become one of the busiest on the East End.

Thankfully, kayaking on Lake Montauk has become almost as popular as fishing. A small number of put-ins exists along the harbor's shores, my favorite of which sits on the eastern side along East Lake Drive. Launching there puts the whole of Lake Montauk and its attractions at your disposal.

USGS Quadrangles
MONTAUK POINT (NY)

13 **DESCRIPTION** Although launching from the beach on East Lake Drive puts you in the water near the

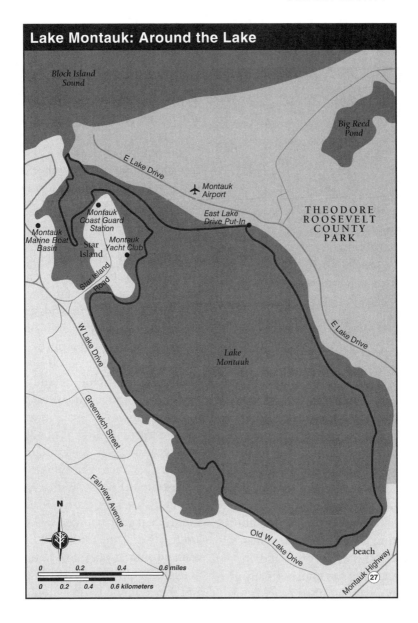

Lake Montauk: Around the Lake

Block Island
Sound

Big Reed
Pond

E Lake Drive

Montauk
Airport

East Lake
Drive Put-In

THEODORE
ROOSEVELT
COUNTY
PARK

Montauk
Coast Guard
Station

Montauk
Marine Boat
Basin

Star
Island

Montauk
Yacht Club

Star Island Road

W Lake Drive

E Lake Drive

Lake
Montauk

Greenwich Street

Fairview Avenue

N

Old W Lake Drive

beach

Montauk Highway 27

| 0 | 0.2 | 0.4 | 0.6 miles |

| 0 | 0.2 | 0.4 | 0.6 kilometers |

northern end of the harbor, there's a lot of kayak-worthy water to the south. Follow the eastern shore in that direction, and one of the first things you'll notice is the quiet. Sure, there are boats in the area. And Jet Skis. And water-skiers. With most marinas and docks near the harbor's entrance,

though, the remainder of the harbor is remarkably peaceful.

The quiet is also quite surprising considering the number of homes that line the harbor. Almost the entire eastern shore, from the put-in at East Lake Drive to the southernmost corner, is lined with houses. It really isn't

Around the Lake

Level	2B
Distance	6.7 miles around
Time	3 hours
Navigable months	Year-round
Hazards	Boat traffic, especially at its northern end
Portages	None
Rescue access	Easy
Tidal conditions	Any
Scenery	B–B+

necessary given the laid-back attitude of the residents, but paddling a bit offshore can help alleviate the distractions of civilization from a serene and calming paddle. If you're paddling anywhere but right next to the beach, though, take note of any buoys marked POSTED or CLAM FARM. These notices mark the boundaries of ongoing shellfish-restoration projects, which should be given a wide berth whenever possible.

A small marina with some large boats sits 0.75 mile south of the put-in, marking the approximate halfway point of the eastern shore. Paddle 1 mile farther and the houses finally give way to some undisturbed beachfront, at least for a short while anyway. Soon a small town beach pops up, replete with moored boats and personal watercraft or paddleboarders during the summer months. Once you pass them, your compass should finally swing north as you begin to head up the western shore of the harbor.

Although this shoreline is just as developed as its opposite, its houses are fairly well hidden by beach grass and landscaping shrubs. While this may not be the most pristine environment in which to paddle, the effect is welcoming. In fact, the beach heather and marsh elder growing in some spots is absolutely beautiful.

Keep hugging the shore and you'll come to a small, sandy spit of land less than 1 mile from the town beach at the south end of the harbor. Skirt around it to reach a decent-sized cove lying farther south. Amazingly, most of the cove has remained undeveloped, rimmed with spartina grass, beach heather, and some phragmites reeds instead. Phragmites notwithstanding, the cove most likely resembles what the whole of the harbor once looked like, long before real estate agents began selling off plots of land.

You may find it difficult to pay much attention to the plants and wildlife along the beaches beyond the southern cove, since Star Island and its immense yacht clubs loom in the distance to the north. With a narrow causeway blocking the western route, you must paddle counterclockwise around the island. Of course, this puts you and your kayak into a potential maelstrom of fishing boats, trawlers, and megayachts. Truth be told, though, this really is one of the most fascinating places to paddle.

GPS COORDINATES

Put-in/take-out
N41° 04.267' W71° 55.228'
Tide station
Montauk Harbor Entrance, NY
N41° 04.500' W71° 56.202'

As you round the southeastern tip of Star Island, look for the sprawling resort and marina of the Montauk Yacht Club, complete with its very own lighthouse. Some of the most handsome boats you may ever see are usually docked just beyond the resort's beach. Continue past the yacht club's grounds and round the tip of Star Island, and you'll be paddling past the Montauk Coast Guard Station, with its stark white cutter poised for a quick sprint out of the harbor if needed. To the south and southwest sit more marinas, restaurants, and a bar or two, although the real excitement is to the north.

This section of the harbor, the Montauk Marine Boat Basin, is where some world-renowned charter boats operate from, catching everything from striped bass to tuna, swordfish to shark. It is also where dozens of commercial fishing boats and trawlers operate from, loading supplies and unloading their catch throughout the fishing season. On any given day here, you may see a thresher shark or a mako hanging from a scale on the dock, a charter boat packed with paying customers, or a rusty trawler tying up, its hold filled with the day's catch. Factor in the amazing seafood restaurants alongside the docks, and the boat basin may be hard to leave.

When you do decide to leave the basin, the harbor's inlet is just a few paddle strokes to the north. It may not be prudent to kayak through the inlet at times, however, given how crowded it can get. Picture the scene in *Jaws* where all of the townsfolk are in their boats zigzagging around the harbor, and you'll have a fairly good picture of what the inlet can look like during

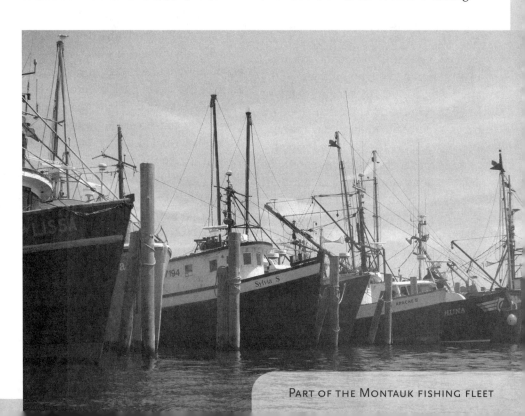

PART OF THE MONTAUK FISHING FLEET

busy summer days. Paddling between the jetties toward Block Island Sound definitely requires steady maneuvering and solid boat skills, as well as suitable weather conditions. Instead of going this route, you can round Star Island, clockwise this time, to gain access to the harbor's eastern side once again. From there, the small beach from which you launched is only slightly more than 1 mile away.

◇ **SHUTTLE DIRECTIONS** To get to the put-in on the eastern side of Montauk Harbor, take NY 27 (Montauk Highway) to the village of Montauk. Pass through the town and continue east 2 miles. Turn left onto East Lake Drive and continue north another 2 miles. Look for a small dirt turnoff opposite the Little Reed Pond parking area. Park there and carry your boat down the short path to the water.

14 LAKE RONKONKOMA

◇ **OVERVIEW** Lake Ronkonkoma is Long Island's largest freshwater lake, sitting right in its center near the towns of Smithtown, Brookhaven, and Islip. The lake's original name, *Raconkamuck,* means "The Boundary Fishing Place," although it most likely referred to the boundaries among the local Nissequogue, Setauket, Secatogue, and Unkechaug tribes and not the modern-day towns. Ronkonkoma is a kettle lake, formed by a retreating glacier. It has extremely deep sections of up to 65 feet, but most of the lake is much more shallow.

While the lake has a rather unremarkable history (settled by Native Americans, purchased by Europeans, colonized and developed, and turned into a resort area), it has nonetheless taken on an aura of mystery and legend. Perhaps it's the lake's depth that has spawned some of the many bizarre and frightening stories. Or maybe its murky waters are the source. There's also its close connection to the Native American people who once inhabited its shores. Whatever the reason, the range of tall tales that have sprung up is widespread and enduring.

One of the earliest legends of the lake started in the late 1800s, when large numbers of tourists and vacationers came to Ronkonkoma seeking out the allegedly miraculous healing powers of its waters. Another story involves an inlet that led to the lake from the Atlantic; supposedly, pirates used this opening to gain access to the lake, where they would hide their treasures. The yarns take a wide leap from there, describing schools of piranha, a deadly whirlpool that sucks people and boats down from the center of the lake, and an underwater tunnel that connects the lake to Long Island Sound. Some tales even describe the lake as bottomless.

While many people hold on to these stories and tell and retell them over and over again, one stands out above the rest: the story of the Lady of the Lake.

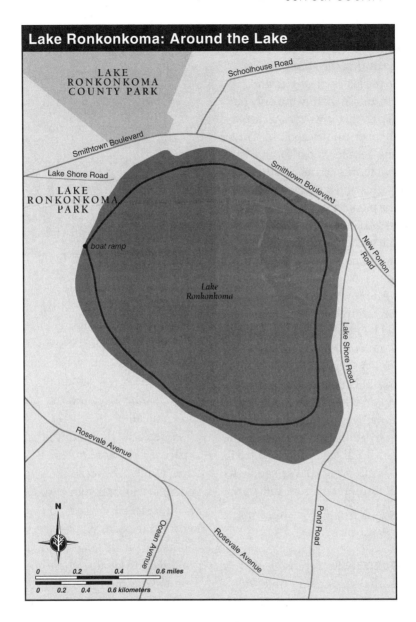

Lake Ronkonkoma: Around the Lake

LAKE RONKONKOMA COUNTY PARK

Schoolhouse Road

Smithtown Boulevard

Lake Shore Road

LAKE RONKONKOMA PARK

Smithtown Boulevard

boat ramp

New Portion Road

Lake Ronkonkoma

Lake Shore Road

Rosevale Avenue

N

Ocean Avenue

Rosevale Avenue

Pond Road

0   0.2   0.4   0.6 miles

0   0.2   0.4   0.6 kilometers

As most Long Islanders have likely heard it, a young Native American princess rises from the depths of the lake each summer to grab a young man and pull him under water. What sent the princess to the lake's bottom depends on who's telling the story, but most versions say she intentionally drowned herself out of grief over a lost love or in protest of an arranged marriage. Many believers in the story cite historical records that lend truth to the claim that one young man drowns in Lake Ronkonkoma each summer; naysayers counter that such fatalities aren't unusual on account of the lake's size and heavy use during the summer.

While the lake's mysteries are intriguing, they're hardly the only reason Ronkonkoma is worth a visit. Recreational opportunities abound. Three swimming beaches, a park with basketball and tennis courts, another with baseball fields and a playground, and numerous picnic areas line the shore. Ice-boating takes place on its surface during the winter months. Fishing for bass, bluegill, pumpkinseed, perch, and carp (and maybe piranha?) is hugely popular. And rowboats, canoes, and kayaks frequently float the lake's waters.

Should you want to paddle Lake Ronkonkoma or try your luck fishing from your kayak for some of its largemouth bass, head no farther than the boat ramp on its western shore, maintained by the New York State Department of Environmental Conservation. You'll easily be able to reach any part of the 0.6-mile-wide lake or paddle its 2-mile circumference from this ramp.

USGS Quadrangles CENTRAL ISLIP (NY), PATCHOGUE (NY)

14 **DESCRIPTION** Because Lake Ronkonkoma is less than 1 mile wide and 2 miles around, you can see the whole of it when standing at the foot of the ramp you're launching from. Thus, with little distance to travel and few paddling options to choose from, your only real decision is whether to travel the lake's perimeter clockwise or counterclockwise. And even then, there's no such thing as the wrong choice.

Around the Lake

Level	1A
Distance	1.9 miles around
Time	1.5 hours
Navigable months	March–December
Hazards	Underwater debris
Portages	None
Rescue access	Easy
Tidal conditions	Spring-fed—not affected by tides
Scenery	B

If you're starting your trip by heading left (north), you'll first be paddling off a lakeshore that is heavily wooded. Red maple and willow trees abound here, as the soil is saturated with fresh water. Paddle just a few hundred feet more and all of those trees will be gone, replaced by a sandy beach that is part of Lake Ronkonkoma County Park. While this would seem to be a good place to land your kayak, doing so is against park rules. So you'll have to continue paddling past the park's ball fields, picnic tables, and playground and look elsewhere should you want to stop and rest a bit.

Stay close to shore as you leave the park behind, and you may be able to catch a glimpse of a unique Lake

GPS COORDINATES

Put-in/take-out
N40° 49.767' W73° 07.718'

Ronkonkoma feature. Because the lake's water level fluctuates so much with rising and falling groundwater levels (it seems to have been quite high for the past few years), you may find yourself paddling over sections of drowned roadways or parking lots, and you may even see a section of guardrail or two. At the very least, you'll be paddling alongside a stand of trees whose bases are completely submerged, much like the mangrove trees of tropical climates.

The lakeshore will begin to curve eastward as you paddle past the large and partially sunken parking lot of the once-popular Bavarian Inn restaurant. Long closed, the building has obviously seen better days. Just beyond the derelict inn, however, sits a lively establishment that's been going strong for decades. The Parsnip Pub serves great food and drinks, and its deck affords great views of the lake. Paddle past the pub on a sunny day, and you'll surely have a few customers call out to you and offer you a drink or two.

The shoreline changes a bit east of the Parsnip Pub, with a small tree-lined bluff rising up from the water that makes landing difficult, if not impossible to accomplish. Such conditions continue for the next mile or so, with nearby Portion Road and eventually Lake Shore Road running parallel to the top of the tiny bluff. The road noise will be somewhat loud along this stretch of shore, even with the ever-present maple and willow trees acting as a barrier.

After paddling about halfway around the lake (0.75 mile), you'll reach the Windows on the Lake catering hall, where, if you're lucky, a wedding or other large party will be going on. Of course, you should be respectful of the partygoers. That said, it's always fun trying to get your picture taken and put in an unsuspecting guest's album.

Head just 0.3 mile farther south to reach another small beach. Unlike the first one you paddled past, this beach allows boats to land, making it a great rest stop if necessary. If not, forge on as the lakeshore curves west, and you'll be treated to a scene much more natural than any you've just paddled past. The roads will have left the lakeside, the bluff will have risen a bit higher, and most of the waterfront houses will be hidden from your view.

Thankfully, you'll be paddling along this serene shoreline for the last 0.75 mile of your trip, although there is one small break where another town beach sits. Otherwise, you'll be able to finish your trip around Lake Ronkonkoma reveling in its natural beauty.

⟡ **SHUTTLE DIRECTIONS** To get to your put-in at the Department of Environmental Conservation Lake Access site, take the Long Island Expressway (I-495) to Exit 59N (Ocean Avenue). Take Ocean Avenue north 0.7 mile before it meets Rosevale Avenue. Pick up Rosevale Avenue and continue north another 0.7 mile. Turn right onto Victory Drive and head east 0.2 mile. The access site is at the end of Victory Drive.

15   LLOYD HARBOR

✧ **OVERVIEW** Along Long Island's moneyed North Shore, between Cold Spring and Huntington harbors, lies the stunning body of water called Lloyd Harbor. It runs west to east, almost connecting the two neighboring harbors and all but separating the peninsula of Lloyd Neck from the mainland. With a great deal of prime real estate along its shores and throughout the village of the same name, Lloyd Harbor has long been home to some of Long Island's wealthiest people. (One of the estates for which Lloyd Harbor is famous, Oheka Castle, helped inspire F. Scott Fitzgerald to write *The Great Gatsby*.)

Lloyd Harbor wasn't always such a fashionable place, however. Nor was it always called Lloyd Harbor. In fact, the area's original inhabitants, the Matinecock Native Americans, called it *Caumsett*, or "Place by a Sharp Rock," likely referring to the large erratics, or boulders, that lie off the east coast of the Lloyd Neck Peninsula. After purchasing the land from the natives for only three coats and shirts, a couple of pairs of shoes, six knives, and a handful of wampum, the Europeans renamed it Horse Neck since they mainly used it as a place for their horses to graze.

Then, in 1684, a man by the name of James Lloyd came to Horse Neck and became its sole owner. He quickly renamed the area "Manor of Queen's Village" and began leasing it out to interested farmers. Upon his death, James's son Henry inherited the land and built a house on part of what is now Caumsett State Park. The Lloyd family, having established roots in the area, continued to pass the land down

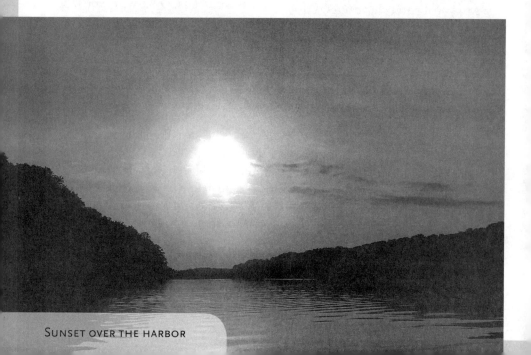

SUNSET OVER THE HARBOR

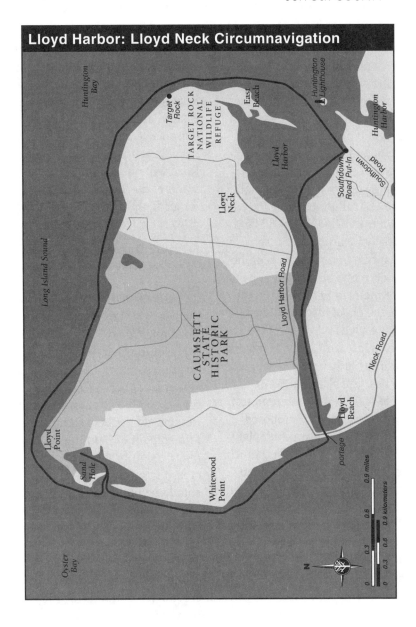

Lloyd Harbor: Lloyd Neck Circumnavigation

from one generation to the next until the late 1800s. In that time, a steamboat ferry dock had been built along the causeway that leads to the peninsula, a tidal mill was constructed to service the area, and the newly renamed village of Lloyd Neck officially seceded from Queens County and became part of Huntington Town. Throughout all of these new developments, though, Lloyd Neck remained mostly undisturbed, with only a small population of landowners living within its borders.

All of that began to change with the dawn of the new century as the country's rich and famous began to seek out places to build luxurious estates. With both natural beauty and exclusivity, Lloyd Neck proved the perfect place for the elite to settle. Grand mansions with sprawling lawns and immense gardens began to pop up across the peninsula and on the mainland as Long Island entered its Gold Coast heyday. Still, the area remained relatively uncrowded, with only a small population of full-time residents. In fact, when the village of Lloyd Harbor was officially incorporated in 1926, its rural appeal and protection of the area's undeveloped land were top on the list of motivating factors.

While the era of the Gold Coast estates has ended and many of the area's wealthiest families have moved on, Lloyd Harbor has managed to retain much of its original appeal. More than a few large-scale development projects have been squelched, the proposed construction of a nuclear power plant was successfully fought off, and much once-private land has been set aside as parkland, forever preserved as open space. Two of those parks, Caumsett State Historic Park and the Target Rock National Wildlife Refuge, are indeed two of the area's treasures.

Although most of us can't afford to buy an estate in Lloyd Harbor, we can easily paddle along its waters. The beach on the causeway leading to Lloyd Neck is a great place to set out on a circumnavigation of the peninsula, as long as you have a Town of Huntington parking permit. Otherwise, look to the shoulder of Lloyd Harbor Road along the peninsula's southern shore for a place to park your car and launch a kayak or two. Be very careful,

though, as the village's police are always eager to issue tickets to those who've parked in unauthorized areas. An easier spot, one that is free and legal for everyone, sits on the southeastern end of Lloyd Harbor, near the entrance to Huntington Harbor. This small beach at the end of Southdown Road will put you on the water due south of the Target Rock refuge, poised for a trip up Lloyd Neck's eastern shore or west on Lloyd Harbor itself.

USGS Quadrangles
LLOYD HARBOR (NY)

15 **DESCRIPTION** Launching from the beach at the end of Southdown Road puts you on the water a bit west of the entrance to Huntington Harbor and due south of a long and narrow spit of land that makes up the tip of the Target Rock National Wildlife Refuge. While the boat traffic heading into and out of Huntington Harbor may be significant, the half-mile crossing to the refuge on Lloyd Neck should be pretty easy to accomplish. The area west of the harbor entrance does have quite a few boats floating on their moorings which do require some attention, though their speeds should be fairly slow whenever they are moving and thus, be easy to avoid. If the wind is calm and boat traffic at a minimum during the crossing, the Huntington Lighthouse that sits just beyond the harbor entrance makes a worthy photo stop. (See page 68 for more information on the light.)

Once across the mouth of Lloyd Harbor, keep the sandy beach to your left and you'll soon enter the Target Rock National Wildlife Refuge. While

Lloyd Neck Circumnavigation

Level	2C
Distance	12.4 miles around
Time	5 hours
Navigable months	Year-round
Hazards	Open water, boat traffic
Portages	1
Rescue access	Easy
Tidal conditions	Any (but portage at high tide only)
Scenery	A+

the majority of this 80-acre refuge resides on high and dry ground, with old-growth oak and hickory forests throughout, its 0.5-mile beach provides an excellent place to paddle. If you're paddling here in spring or summer, you'll surely see double-crested cormorants in great numbers. Great blue herons, great egrets, and snowy egrets are also plentiful along the refuge's shores. Slow down some and look a bit more carefully at the rocky beach, and you may see a few piping plovers as well as willets, black-bellied plovers, and sandpipers. Bank swallows, kingfishers, red-tailed hawks, and ospreys frequent the shores as well. In fact, a most unusual osprey nest can be found near the southern tip of the refuge, atop an old, abandoned brick structure.

Paddle here during the winter and you'll see a completely different assortment of wildlife along the shore. Gone will be the wading birds, replaced by waterfowl. Black ducks usually predominate here, while long-tailed ducks, scaups, buffleheads, goldeneyes, and red-breasted mergansers round out the mix.

If birds don't interest you, perhaps the bluefish, striped bass, and blackfish will. Or maybe New York's only cactus species, the prickly pear, will draw your attention growing along the shore. Then there are the harbor seals that play among the refuge's waves during the winter. I even paddled past a small sea turtle feeding a few hundred feet off the beach one fall day.

While the shore remains completely undeveloped within Target Rock's boundaries, it changes a bit after 1.7 miles. You'll notice that once it begins to curve to the west, some houses appear along the bluffs, with some boat docks breaking up the shore in the distance. A good number of decent-sized rocks also begin to appear in the water off the beach at this point. Legend has it that the largest rock found here was used by the British army for target practice during both the Revolutionary War and the War of 1812. Though unsubstantiated, the story did provide the refuge with its name.

The beach continues to curve for the next mile until you are paddling almost due west, with Lloyd Neck on

GPS COORDINATES

Put-in/take-out
N40° 54.476' W73° 26.354'
Tide station
Lloyd Harbor Entrance,
Huntington Bay, NY
N40° 54.600' W73° 25.902'

your left and Long Island Sound on your right. The shores of Connecticut, just across the sound, can appear deceivingly close on clear, sunny days. They are, in fact, about 5 miles away. Closer, though, are the iconic bluffs of Caumsett State Park. Travel past the few remaining houses sitting on the water's edge, beyond the last small jetties breaking up the shore's straight run, and you'll be soon be paddling in the shadows of these bluffs. Indeed, the park's boundary is only 1.5 miles from the "target rock."

While cruising along Target Rock may have given you a chance to study the area's wildlife, paddling along Caumsett's shores provides a lesson in geology. Look closely at the 30-foot-high cliffs on the park's beach, and you'll find sediments that are more than 65 million years old. In fact, Caumsett is one of the few places on Long Island where you can see such a formation that dates back to the Cretaceous Period. Also note the dozens of large rocks that sit on Caumsett's beach: like the "target rock" from earlier in your trip, these boulders, or erratics, are evidence of Long Island's glacial history. Amazingly, glaciers picked up these huge rocks far to our north and carried them great distances before depositing them on the North Shore. Because they are composed of a wide variety of minerals, these erratics help make Caumsett's shoreline "a veritable geologist's supermarket," as Robert Villani, author of *Long Island: A Natural History,* puts it.

Caumsett's classic bluffs shrink after 2 miles, leaving a low-lying and marshy area along the northernmost

tip of Lloyd Neck. Round this point, known as Lloyd Point, and you'll be heading almost due south, directly toward Cold Spring Harbor. With 5 miles of paddle strokes already behind you, you may be feeling a bit tired and ready to head for home. Or perhaps the wind and tides are now conspiring against you and slowing your forward progress. If either of these scenarios is the case, you may want to forge straight ahead and make your way to the Lloyd Harbor portage (itself about 3 miles distant). If you do have the time and energy, though, a short excursion into the area known by locals as the "Sand Hole" is definitely worth your while.

About 0.75 mile south of Lloyd Point, the Sand Hole is protected from the wind and waves by an entrance that is both narrow and shallow. While not much of a challenge for kayakers, these conditions can prove a bit tricky for powerboaters who may also be trying to enter the great anchoring spot. Should you be entering the channel at the same time as one of these bigger vessels, be kind and give it the right of way, remembering that there is more than enough room once inside for everyone.

Once you're inside the Sand Hole, most of the powerboaters will tend to anchor near the deeper water and beaches on the left (west) side. Hugging the opposite shore allows you to avoid them and also brings you to a maze of small channels that spread throughout the fairly extensive salt marsh found there. In fact, you may find yourself spending at least an hour or two exploring the twists and turns that wind between the mats of peat and stands of spartina grass. Enjoy yourself, but keep an eye on both your watch and the tide. If you don't, you could end up wading through mud that is wider and deeper than you would like.

Soon either time or tide will force you to leave the Sand Hole and continue your trip south around Lloyd Neck. Follow its steeply sloped shore for another mile, and you'll reach another turning point, known as Whitewood Point. If you look straight ahead as you turn your kayak to the southeast, your portage spot over the Lloyd Neck causeway should come into view. Although this last stretch of water, between Whitewood Point and the portage, is only 1 mile long, it's quite enjoyable, as the water views of Cold Spring Harbor to the south and Centre Island to the west are stunning.

Also worth noting are the houses overlooking your path, most of which will seem to have grown in both size and extravagance from earlier in your trip. Take special note of the brick house at the water's edge, immediately before the rocky barrier along the causeway—the best spot for a portage is just south of its iron fence. Paddle past the home's beachfront, a few feet south of its fence, and hop out of your boat onto a small stretch of sand between the rocks. You need to carry your boat over the rocks and across the street at this point. A paddling partner and/or a good set of wheels can make this task much easier. Once you've made it across, just follow the short trail between the trees and through the marsh, and you can put in again on Lloyd Harbor and continue the last leg of your circumnavigation.

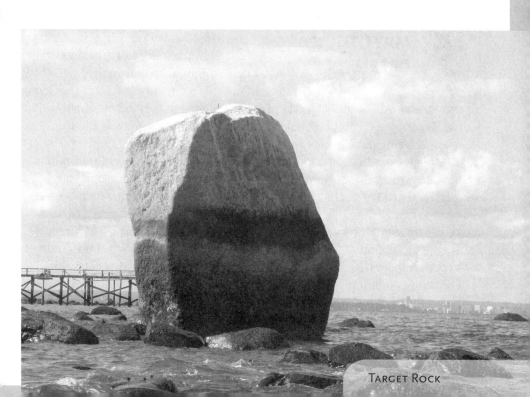

Target Rock

Lloyd Harbor boasts another marsh that is worthy of exploration, due south of your portage spot. You may choose to skip this one, though, since you have more than 9 miles of paddling behind you and 3 miles still to come. There is no shame in doing so, considering the beauty you'll experience in the harbor itself. There is almost no development at all along the long, narrow harbor's length. Instead, its waters are bordered by continuous forests of oak, maple, locust, and chestnut. Stay observant and you'll likely see a kingfisher or two flitting among the trees or a red-tailed hawk soaring overhead. Few, if any, powerboats venture into the harbor's shallower waters, and only at its mouth do any boats float on a mooring. This is a splendid place to end a successful circumnavigation. Once you're through the harbor, head to the southeast and you'll reach the beach from which you launched 0.7 mile later.

✧ **SHUTTLE DIRECTIONS** To get to the Lloyd Harbor put-in, take the Northern State Parkway to Exit 40N (NY 110). Take NY 110 north for 5.6 miles into the village of Huntington. Turn left onto Main Street (NY 25A) and take the first right onto Wall Street. Continue north on Wall Street 0.6 mile before turning left onto Southdown Road. Follow Southdown Road until it ends at the water 3 miles later. Park anywhere along the side of the road, and carry your boat over the rocks to the water's edge.

16 MATTITUCK CREEK

✧ **OVERVIEW** Although Long Island's long and convoluted coastline makes for a sea-kayaking paradise, its North Shore stretch from Mt. Sinai to Orient Point is almost completely devoid of any places to paddle. Thankfully, the only major break along this section of coast, known as Mattituck Creek, provides a superb option for those looking to get out on the water.

The Native Americans who once inhabited the Mattituck area surely recognized the value of their land, for they named it *Mattatuck,* or "Great Creek." The name is also thought to have meant "Land of Few Trees," perhaps in reference to the vast salt marshes that once existed along the creek. Either way, the natives were obviously fond of their 2-mile stretch of water, though they did eventually sell it and its adjoining lands to Englishmen from nearby Southold for the then-steep sum of 7 pounds of wampum.

As with most of their other landholdings, the Europeans then began parceling out this new purchase to interested settlers. Farms, a church, tavern, and an inn popped up almost immediately after that. A couple of centuries later, a school, a branch of the Long Island Rail Road, a post office, and two factories came, leaving Mattituck ready to enter the 20th century. But it wasn't until a yacht club and four

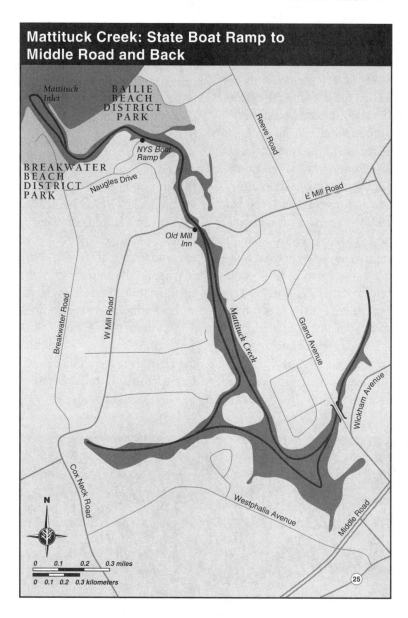

Mattituck Creek: State Boat Ramp to Middle Road and Back

Mattituck Inlet

BAILIE BEACH DISTRICT PARK

NYS Boat Ramp

BREAKWATER BEACH DISTRICT PARK

Naugles Drive

Reeve Road

E Mill Road

Old Mill Inn

Breakwater Road

W Mill Road

Mattituck Creek

Grand Avenue

Wickham Avenue

Cox Neck Road

Westphalia Avenue

Middle Road

N

0   0.1   0.2   0.3 miles

0   0.1   0.2   0.3 kilometers

25

summer hotels opened that the area's popularity among the boating crowd took hold. Even now, almost a century later, Mattituck has remained an excellent place to tie up one's lines.

Although our boats may be a bit different from the majority of those docked or floating on moorings in the creek, they're still quite welcome in Mattituck's waters. And with the construction of a state boat ramp at its northern end, they can be launched easier than ever. So grab your PFD and paddle, secure your kayak to your car's roof, and head to the "Great Creek." You'll be glad you did.

USGS Quadrangles Mattituck
Hills (NY), Mattituck (NY)

16 **DESCRIPTION** You have only one
decision to make after launching from
the state boat ramp onto Mattituck
Creek: north or south? North brings
you to the mouth of the creek, and
Long Island Sound beyond, in 0.5 mile.
Nothing but an unbroken shoreline
stretches to both the east and west from
there, making it an option few kayakers
take, although I always enjoy poking my
boat out onto open water, even if only to
check on the conditions before heading
into more-protected locations. Your only
other choice, then, is to head south and
explore the rest of Mattituck Creek.

There is little about Mattituck
Creek that screams "nature." In fact,
most of its shores are developed,

taken up by houses and boatyards.
Paddle around the curve in the creek
just south of the boat ramp, and you'll
notice almost immediately that the
quiet serenity of the once-unbroken
shoreline ends and houses begin to
pop up, while just across the creek
the first of many marinas appears.
Although nature-lovers may wince at
the intrusion, boat-lovers will appreciate the variety found here. Mattituck
is home to a large fleet of commercial
boats—fishing-charter boats, trawlers, and lobster boats—and this first
marina is where many of them tie
up their lines. Many private sailboats
and powerboats dock here as well.

Continue south, and 0.5 mile later
you'll come to a large red building on
the right. If it seems that the building is sitting on top of the water, it is.

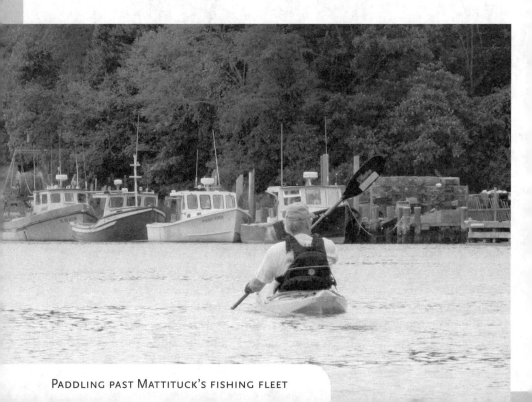

PADDLING PAST MATTITUCK'S FISHING FLEET

State Boat Ramp to Middle Road and Back

Level	1B
Distance	7 miles round-trip
Time	3–4 hours
Navigable months	Year-round (but may freeze in winter)
Hazards	Boat traffic
Portages	None
Rescue access	Easy
Tidal conditions	Any
Scenery	B

Currently home to the Old Mill Inn, it was originally built as a tidal mill in the early 1800s by a man named Samuel Cox. It operated as such for many years before it was converted into a popular tavern in the early 1900s. If you could paddle underneath the building, you'd see a trapdoor that leads straight to the kitchen. This secret entrance was very useful during Prohibition, when it was used to smuggle liquor into the building. With the repeal of Prohibition, the building cleaned up its act a bit by adding a restaurant. This new enterprise proved very profitable, and the Old Mill Inn has remained an eatery ever since. With a waterfront deck for dining and a dock for patrons' use, the Old Mill Inn caters to the boating community. If you find yourself here in the off-season and you're feeling hungry, paddle up to its dock, tie your kayak to a cleat, and order some great food and drinks. (More info: 631-298-8080; **theoldmillinn.net.**)

Once back on the water, you'll paddle past the last marina before reaching the creek's southernmost end. From here on, only private waterfront homes and their requisite docks line the shores. A half-mile south of the Old Mill Inn, a side arm of the creek provides an additional mile of shoreline to explore. Most maps and charts of the area show its entrance just west of a fairly large island stretching across the creek. In reality, this island is actually quite small—more a cluster of small clumps of dry land. Nevertheless, it's a useful marker for the creek's entrance.

If you choose to paddle the creek's length west, you'll be privy to views much like those on the main creek: private homes and boats sitting at their docks. Head a few hundred feet farther south, however, and look for another side creek along the eastern shore if you're craving something different. The creek does start out in much the same way as its partner on the opposite shore, but with a bit of faith and perseverance and a few paddle strokes, the houses soon give way to a more wooded shoreline. Pass under the Grand Avenue bridge, and before you know it, you'll be paddling down a narrow branch of water lined only with spartina grass, phragmites reeds, and an oak forest. The calls of red-winged blackbirds in the reeds

GPS COORDINATES

Put-in/take-out
N41° 00.820' W72° 33.160'
Tide station
Mattituck Inlet, NY
N41° 00.900' W72° 33.702'

will have replaced the sounds of boat motors, and glimpses of egrets and herons will have taken the place of Grady Whites and Catalinas.

Like all good things, this side trip eventually comes to an end as the creek dead-ends 0.5 mile beyond the small bridge near its entrance. As you have little else to see and no farther to go on Mattituck Creek, your only option here is to head north once again and paddle the 1.5 miles back to the state boat ramp and your car. Of course, you could always stop in for another round at the Old Mill Inn.

◇ **SHUTTLE DIRECTIONS** To get to the DEC boat launch on Mattituck Creek, take NY 25 (Sound Avenue) into the village of Mattituck. Turn left onto Cox Neck Road (right if you're coming from the east), and continue north 0.75 mile. Cox Neck Road will turn sharply to the right before turning into West Mill Road. Continue north on West Mill Road and look for the DEC boat-launch sign after 1.25 miles. Turn right into the parking lot and follow the gravel road to the boat ramp and Mattituck Creek.

---

17 MECOX BAY

◇ **OVERVIEW** Though not as large as Shinnecock Bay, its neighbor to the west, or as popular among the rich and famous as Georgica Pond, to the east, Mecox Bay has managed to become a favorite spot of the East End paddling crowd. Why? They appreciate its 15-plus miles of shoreline. They jump at the chance to experience its scenic beauty. They enjoy exploring its side creeks and coves. They bird-watch. They people-watch. They dig clams. They paddle to the ocean beach and picnic. Basically, kayakers love everything about the bay.

Mecox sits in the center of Watermill, south of Montauk Highway and the landmark that the hamlet was named after. Locals are quite proud of this mill and are quick to point out that it is fully functional to this day.

They also like to brag about their windmill, and the fact that their hamlet is the only one on the South Fork that has both a water mill and a windmill within its borders. As a visitor to Watermill, you will likely take note of both of these structures as you drive through town, but your main reason for coming here is probably to paddle that beautiful bay.

Luckily, this is easy to do. Almost every road that parallels or leads to the bay has a small beach area at its end that can be used as a put-in. Most even have room to park one or two cars (or more if you're parking at Flying Point Beach or Scott Cameron Beach). You need a permit from Southampton Town to use of some of these spots legally, though others are free and open to anyone. The put-in at the end of Bay Avenue is my personal favorite, putting you on the water at the bay's northernmost point, ready to begin an amazing paddle on an even more amazing body of water.

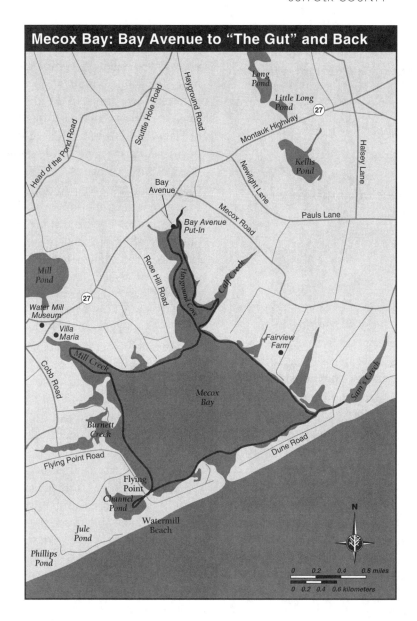

Mecox Bay: Bay Avenue to "The Gut" and Back

USGS Quadrangles
SAG HARBOR (NY)

17 **DESCRIPTION** It's hard to imagine what's in store for you when you launch from the tiny beach at the end of Bay Avenue. The put-in is at the northern-most tip of the northernmost arm of

Mecox Bay, surrounded by 10-foot high reeds of phragmites. From this vantage point, the beauty of the bay is all but hidden from view. While you're prob-ably itching to head south and explore the bay, try putting it off for a few minutes—a small treasure lies waiting just a few paddle strokes to the north.

Bay Avenue to "The Gut" and Back

Level	2B
Distance	8.7 miles round-trip
Time	4 hours
Navigable months	March–November
Hazards	Open water
Portages	None
Rescue access	Easy
Tidal conditions	Any
Scenery	A

Head in that direction and you'll notice that the phragmites-filled shoreline appears to be closing in on you. It is in fact narrowing, funneling you deeper into a quieter stretch of water that feels more streamlike than saltwater. Before long the phragmites will be completely gone, replaced with maple and tupelo trees that block out all but the most persistent rays of sunshine and create a feeling of seclusion that is often hard to obtain from the seat of a sea kayak. Unfortunately, this small creek dead-ends just a bit south of Mecox Road, only a few hundred feet after it began. Don't despair, though, as now you're ready to explore the remainder of Mecox's waters.

Once you've retraced your strokes, you'll again be paddling in the northern section of Mecox Bay, known as Hayground Cove. Hug the eastern shore and you'll likely gaze longingly at the sprawling homes that line the cove. Most seem to be built with cedar shingles, a look that is quite common throughout the Hamptons, and

they seem to grow bigger and more beautiful as you pass them by. Gaze away as you paddle along for the next mile, and soon your attention will be broken by a break in the shoreline. Known as Calf Creek, this arm of Hayground Cove stretches to the northeast for 0.5 mile before it ends, again at Mecox Road. Along the way, Calf Creek passes its own collection of exquisite waterfront homes, each with its own private dock and some form of watercraft (motorized, of course).

Once past Calf Creek, you'll finally leave the protected waters of Hayground Cove and enter the expansive bay, but not before you pass through a bottleneck of sorts where both shores pinch in and form a narrow gap. Although it is now little more than a small island and a shoal that is exposed at low tide, this spit of sand is believed to have crossed from one shore to the other at one time, providing locals with a route that drastically shortened the trip around Mecox Bay.

After your boat skims the shallow bottom on either side of the island, you'll finally be able to see the rest of what Mecox has to offer. One thing that becomes obvious is the lack of houses along the bay's eastern shore. Thankfully, they disappear from view a bit south of the entrance to Hayground Cove. Take note of the last

GPS COORDINATES

Put-in/take-out
N40° 55.198' W72° 20.200'
Tide station
Shinnecock Inlet, NY
N40° 50.200' W72° 28.800'

house you see on the eastern shore, then look just right of it and you'll see another potential put-in, with ample parking for a small handful of cars. A waterfront farm named Fairview comes into view just beyond that, locally famous for a certain reason. I won't tell you exactly what that reason is—check out the farm on Google Earth and see for yourself. Amazing, to say the least!

In addition to its main call to fame, the farm boasts two protected stretches of water, one on either side, that beg to be explored if you have the time. They are separated from the main body of Mecox Bay by thin sandbars, which hide their respective entrances from view just as easily as they protect their waters from the wind and waves. Keep an eye out for two small cuts in the reeds on either side of the farm, and you should be able to find these "secret" entrances. Great egrets and great blue herons seem to enjoy these conditions as much as paddlers do; they're often seen in these two small creeks in good numbers.

Past the farm, a large house designed to look like a Spanish villa (white with a red-tile roof) seems to rise out of the shoreline grasses in the southeast corner of the bay. Head toward the residence, and the entrance to Sam's Creek should open before you. This small opening in the phragmites is incredibly narrow and can be completely blocked off at low tide, but you can portage easily over the small stretch of sand.

Sam's Creek begins as a fairly wide cove but narrows as expected under the bridge that lies straight ahead. (Incidentally, paddlers with a Southampton Town parking permit may park in the lot south of the bridge and use it as a put-in.) Beyond the bridge, Sam's Creek stretches 0.75 mile to the northeast, with a shoreline very similar to that of the main part of the bay.

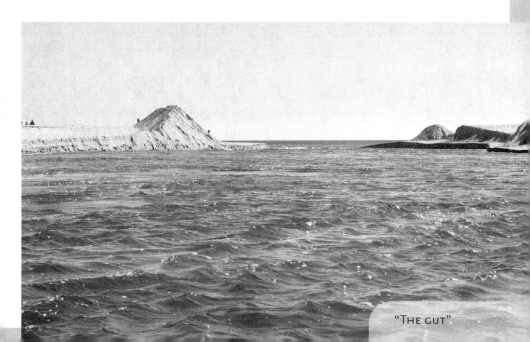

"THE GUT"

Beautiful homes with elaborate yards and landscaping line both sides of the creek, making it more of an architecture-watching site than a bird-watching one, though lucky paddlers may observe some avian species roosting in the trees nearby.

As you leave Sam's Creek and head back to the main bay, paddle along the barrier beach that separates Mecox from the Atlantic, and in 0.75 mile you'll reach a spot where a fierce battle has been raging for centuries. This battle, between man and Mother Nature, began when the native Shinnecock tribe first cut an opening, or *seapoose,* bisecting the beach and allowing salt water to flood into the bay. Their motivation was food: salt water in the bay would create ideal conditions for growing and harvesting shellfish. Although Mother Nature has repeatedly closed the cut, man continues to redig it by hand, animal power, and machine, though our motivations have changed.

Today "the gut," as it is affectionately known, is periodically cut by bulldozers and backhoes to create conditions ideal for fishing, recreational boating, and estuarine-habitat preservation. Whatever the reason for its existence, the gut is a unique and fun place to spend time in, especially on a hot summer day. Jump in, cool off, and ride the tide a bit before continuing your trip around Mecox Bay. Don't paddle too close to the tidal path, though, or you might get caught up in its current and swept out into the Atlantic.

Whereas the gut is evidence of man's fight against Mother Nature, the small pond in Mecox's southwest corner shows what can happen when man leaves things alone. Called Channel Pond, it is almost completely devoid of development. Instead, it is rimmed with phragmites, spartina grass, and other common shoreline plants. Terns, swallows, and egrets are incredibly common on the pond's waters, but

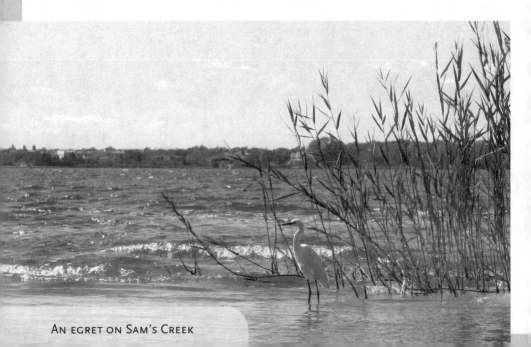

AN EGRET ON SAM'S CREEK

people are not. Chances are you'll have the entirety of its mile-long shoreline to yourself. Pass under the small bridge marking Channel Pond's entrance, and revel in its serenity.

A wooden bulkhead stretches from the entrance to Channel Pond north, leading to yet another extension of Mecox Bay called Burnett Creek. Head west down its waters and you'll gain an additional half-mile of shoreline to explore. Then paddle on and you'll come to what will probably be the last stop on your clockwise trip around Mecox Bay. Once there you should find another stream, called Mill Creek, and a few other points of interest. The first is a relatively unbroken shore to the north. The second is the stunning Villa Maria property, just before Montauk Highway. Built in 1887 as a spiritual retreat, the large estate was recently purchased by a private family who have plans to restore the estate to its prior glory. Finally, Mill Pond lies just beyond Montauk Highway.

Paddle underneath the highway and onto Mill Pond, and you'll likely be amazed at the drastic change in scenery you find. The estuarine environment of Mecox Bay in no way resembles the wooded shore found here. Follow this shore to the right, and you'll come to the mill for which the pond, creek, and town of Watermill are named. You'll also come to the end of the navigable portion of the creek, requiring an about-face.

Once back on the bay, head east along the northern shore until you reach Hayground Cove 1 mile later. From this point, your car is only 0.5 mile to the north.

✧ **SHUTTLE DIRECTIONS** To get to the put-in at the end of Bay Avenue, take NY 27 (Montauk Highway) into the town of Watermill. Look for Bay Avenue just 0.3 mile east of Scuttle Hole Road. Turn onto Bay Avenue and head south until you reach the water.

---

18 MONTAUK POINT

✧ **OVERVIEW** While the village of Montauk signals the end of many people's trips on the South Fork of Long Island, one of the island's most iconic landmarks sits just 5 miles farther at the end of Montauk Highway. Known simply as the Montauk Point Lighthouse, this beloved structure has watched over the easternmost tip of Long Island since George Washington

authorized its construction in 1792. It's the oldest lighthouse in New York State and the fourth oldest in the United States.

Amazingly, when the lighthouse was completed in 1796, the edge of the bluff in front of it was actually 200 feet farther away than it is today. However, the immense erosional forces of the ocean around it have washed a huge amount of sediment away, putting the lighthouse's integrity in danger. Thankfully, control measures—mainly rock walls and terrace plantings—have staved off this erosion, though the

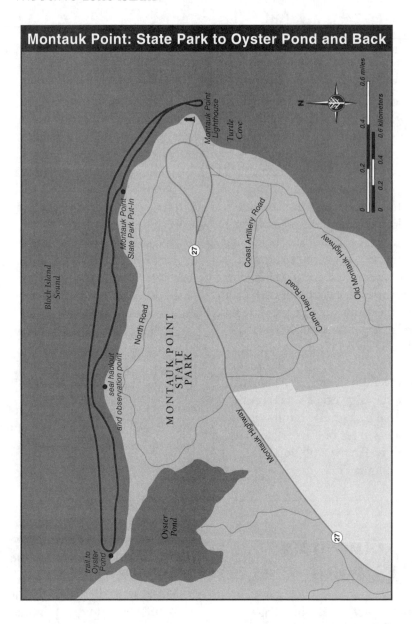

Montauk Point: State Park to Oyster Pond and Back

Montauk Point Lighthouse

Turtle Cove

Montauk Point State Park Put-In

Block Island Sound

Coast Artillery Road

Old Montauk Highway

Camp Hero Road

North Road

seal haulout and observation point

MONTAUK POINT STATE PARK

Montauk Highway

Oyster Pond

trail to Oyster Pond

0.6 miles
0.6 kilometers

strong currents and heavy pounding of the ocean waves are ever-present.

It is these consistently large waves that bring serious surfers to Montauk Point, and it is these same waves that can make the waterway a challenge to paddle. Kayaking here obliges you to deal not only with surf but also with cold water and a rock-strewn beach where the ability to perform surf landings can be a necessity. That said, if conditions are agreeable and your skill level is up to par, Montauk Point can be an amazing place to paddle. It boasts abundant wildlife, its geology is remarkable, and its scenery is simply stunning. One trip here and Montauk will be one of your favorite paddling destinations. It's definitely one of mine.

Unfortunately, launching a kayak at Montauk Point is something of a chore unless you have a permit from the state to drive on the beach. If so, you can simply drive down to the water in front of the snack bar and unload your boat and gear before parking in the lot above. If not, you'll just have to carry everything down to the water—a task made much simpler with a partner and/or a sturdy kayak cart.

USGS Quadrangles
MONTAUK POINT (NY)

18 **DESCRIPTION** Paddle off the rocky beach on the north side of Montauk Point State Park, and you'll be floating on a body of water known as Block Island Sound. You probably won't be able to see Block Island from here, as it's more than 14 miles to the northeast, though you should have a good view of the iconic Montauk Point Lighthouse in the distance over your right shoulder. From this section of beach, known as Montauk's "False Point," the lighthouse sits just 0.5 mile along the rock-strewn coast, roughly marking the point where Block Island Sound ends and the Atlantic Ocean begins. In fact, if you paddle to the lighthouse and beyond, you'll be riding the ocean swell as it rolls toward the Ditch Plains shore.

Head west from the beach and you'll have less of a swell to contend with as you paddle along the point's northern shore. This will give you a chance to slow down and marvel at the beauty of the area. Look to the north and nothing

State Park to Oyster Pond and Back

Level	4B
Distance	4.8 miles round-trip
Time	2 hours
Navigable months	Year-round
Hazards	Tidal currents, waves, rocks
Portages	None
Rescue access	Limited
Tidal conditions	Any
Scenery	A+

but fishing boats and open water is visible. Look to the south along the beach and you'll find a rugged, undeveloped stretch of sand and rock.

The small rocks on the beach and the larger boulders, or erratics, in the water are remnants of the glacial activity that formed Long Island thousands of years ago. In fact, the Montauk Peninsula represents the easternmost tip of the Ronkonkoma Moraine, which was created when one glacier stopped its advance and deposited the sediment it had accumulated at its base. Paddle just offshore here and you'll clearly see the result of this geologic activity.

Continue west, avoiding the erratics that may be sitting just under the

GPS COORDINATES

Put-in/take-out
N41° 04.595' W71° 51.764'
Tide station
Montauk Point, NY
N41° 04.302' W71° 51.402'

water's surface, and the shore begins a graceful curve to the south. Sands in an amazing assortment of colors cover this stretch of beach, although they may not be visible from your current vantage point. Taking their colors from the rocks they were weathered from, these sand grains are yet another end product of the glacial activity that acted upon the island long ago. Whether or not you can see the sands from the water, you can definitely see the 10- to 20-foot bluffs that rise from the water's edge. Though not as dramatic as the bluffs on the peninsula's ocean side, they do add to the natural beauty of this shoreline.

After 1 mile of paddling along the bluffs and rocky beach, you'll reach a cluster of larger rocks jutting out of the water near a small point of land. Many of them will be easily visible from the cockpit of a kayak, but a few others will likely remain submerged and hidden. For this reason, you may want to stay well offshore of this area as you round the point and continue your westward heading. But take a good look at the largest of these rocks as you pass by— they're a popular seal haul-out during the winter and spring months. You should also see a seal-observation platform atop the nearest bluff on shore. If you're lucky enough to see some seals while you are paddling here, be mindful of their sensitive nature and stay as far away from them as possible. Despite their inquisitiveness and puppy-dog-like faces, seals are wild animals and should be left alone.

The beach forms another arc west of the observation platform and curves slowly toward the next point of land,

Shagwong Point. The steep bluffs that lined the shore east of the platform will have softened along this new beach, creating a dunelike barrier to the land behind them. Part of Theodore Roosevelt County Park, this land contains a gorgeous freshwater pond. Known as Oyster Pond, it is usually cut off from the salt water you're paddling by the steep beach that makes up its northern shore. However, this beach is sometimes blown open by strong storms and heavy wave action, allowing some salt water and fresh water to mix. This has the welcome effect of creating conditions ideal for cultivating oysters in the pond. If you have time, land your boat on the beach here and take a good look at the pond. You may even choose to portage your boat onto its waters and paddle around its 2-mile circumference. You won't be disappointed.

If you plan to paddle to Shagwong Point from here, continue hugging the beach as it curves to the northwest and follow it 0.5 more miles. But if you want to paddle to the lighthouse and get a good look at it from the water, turn your boat around and head back east. You'll reach False Point in 2 miles and will pass your launch site just beyond that. Once you've passed it, you'll probably notice that the water has become a bit rougher. Of course, you'll be getting closer and closer to the Atlantic Ocean, so this is to be expected. The shoreline will also appear a bit craggier than before, a result of the increased erosion from the wind and waves. You'll pass in front of the state park's main building, which houses its restaurant and gift shop, and a small sitting area where some park-goers will probably be watching you through the binoculars mounted there.

Finally, you'll reach the lighthouse itself. At its base is a large wall of rocks, designed to dissipate the ocean waves' energy and lessen erosion. They can also easily break apart a kayak, so stay well offshore as you round the light. You'll also get a good look at the terracing that was done on the cliff below the light, which has proved extremely effective at preventing further erosion. Most importantly, you'll see the lighthouse as it was meant to be seen: from the water. One hundred ten feet tall, not counting the height of the bluff it stands on, the light truly towers above you. Its white paint stands out brightly against the blue sky. And its flashing light easily draws your attention. Indeed, kayaking below the lighthouse is a memorable experience.

After you've reached the light, you can continue around the point and paddle Montauk's southern shore on the Atlantic Ocean. If so, you'll first be kayaking in Turtle Cove, a small cove popular with the surfing crowd.

Beyond it, almost 2 miles of unde-veloped beach stretch along an area known as Ditch Plains. Paddle along the shore here and you'll be privy to some of the most spectacular coastal scenery anywhere on Long Island. Steep bluffs, huge erratics, and large hoodoos exist almost as far as you can see, while the ocean and its waves crash onto the beach with a constant rhythm. After just a few paddle strokes here, you'll realize why some consider this the prettiest spot on the island.

If you don't have time to kayak the peninsula's south shore, or if conditions are too rough to venture any farther past the lighthouse, then simply turn your bow around and head back along the northern shore to the beach along False Point. You'll have only 0.5 mile to paddle before you reach your take-out.

◇ **SHUTTLE DIRECTIONS** To get to the put-in in Montauk Point State Park, take Montauk Highway (NY 27) east to its end. Park in the lot closest to the snack bar, and carry your boat and gear down the path to the water on its left.

---

19 MORICHES BAY

◇ **OVERVIEW** Only 8 miles wide and less than 2 miles long, with water that is shallow and well protected, Moriches Bay is one of best paddling spots along Long Island's South Shore. Truth be told, the bay is actually a lagoon, formed by melting glaciers and

rising sea levels and blocked off from the Atlantic by barrier beaches. Fire Island makes up the western portion of that barrier, while the West Hampton Dunes form the eastern portion. Together they help guard the small islands, spartina marshes, and sandy beaches scattered throughout the bay.

Anyone who has driven a boat or paddled a kayak on Moriches Bay remarks about how shallow it is. Depths around the bay average only

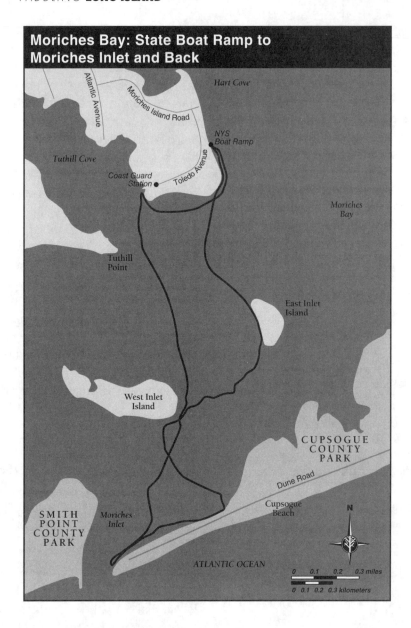

Moriches Bay: State Boat Ramp to Moriches Inlet and Back

about 6 feet, while the Long Island Intracoastal Waterway that cuts through it, connecting the Great South Bay to Shinnecock Bay, is only slightly deeper than that. As a result, larger boats must exercise caution when navigating the bay and usually must stay within the channel markers or risk running aground. Luckily for us, 6 feet is more than enough water to float a kayak. As a result, we paddlers can have most of Moriches Bay to ourselves.

Moriches Bay may just be a sea kayaker's paradise. Because of its size, most of it is well suited to a day trip. The Fire Island barrier beach, on the bay's southwestern side, is just one of its many superb kayaking destinations, with almost 6 miles of undeveloped shoreline begging to be explored. The beachfront community on the West Hampton Dunes side is also an enjoyable place to paddle and do a bit of people-watching. On calm days, the Moriches Inlet, created by a storm in 1931, can be a popular destination, just as nearby Cupsogue Beach is the place to paddle with the local seal population on winter days. To the north numerous tidal creeks await, with Seatuck, Hart, and Tuthill coves and the Forge River rounding out the exciting paddling possibilities.

As we kayakers know all too well, great paddling destinations don't always go hand-in-hand with easy water access. Thankfully, Moriches Bay has both. New York State has constructed a beautiful boat launch next to the Moriches Coast Guard Station that is free and open to anyone interested in getting on the water. It has a small beach and a concrete ramp for launching boats, a short but lovely boardwalk for taking a stroll, and enough parking to accommodate large groups.

USGS Quadrangles
EASTPORT (NY), MORICHES (NY)

19 **DESCRIPTION** If you're planning to visit the barrier beaches along Moriches Bay's southern shore, you'll first have to hug the beach and paddle past the marked boundary of the Moriches Coast Guard Station, at the tip of the peninsula. Note the signs and metal fencing around the property, and try not to get too close, even if you're curious. That said, I like to check out

State Boat Ramp to Moriches Inlet and Back

Level	3A
Distance	5.4 miles round-trip
Time	2 hours
Navigable months	Year-round
Hazards	Open water, tidal currents, boat traffic
Portages	None
Rescue access	Limited
Tidal conditions	3 hours before or after high tide
Scenery	A

which, if any, boats are floating in the station's small dock area, and I often take a quick side trip around the peninsula to see for myself. Should you do the same, you may be able to see some of the Coast Guard's fleet tied up at the dock or tucked away in the boat garages built in to the station house. It's always reassuring for kayakers to see that the Coast Guard is there and ready should we need any help.

Once you're ready to move on, look south across the bay and you should see two fairly large islands formed from the spoils of dredging ahead of you. Neither one is very far off—

GPS COORDINATES

Put-in/take-out
N40° 47.421' W72° 44.706'
Tide station
Moriches Inlet, NY
N40° 45.900' W72° 45.198'

0.7 mile or so—though you'll have to paddle around the westernmost island, appropriately named West Inlet Island, to reach Moriches Inlet. Aim for the 0.4-mile gap between it and its partner, East Inlet Island, and head straight toward the West Hampton Dunes barrier beach. Alternately, you can aim slightly to the west and paddle to West Inlet Island, where terns, herons, snowy and great egrets, glossy ibises, and great black-backed gulls are known to nest. If you visit the island during nesting season, the noise of its many avian species can be deafening. Of course, you shouldn't disturb any birds that may be trying to raise a family on the sand. Instead, maintain a safe distance and don't linger too long.

After you've passed both Inlet Islands, you'll have only 0.4 more miles of paddling before you reach the barrier beach. Assuming you've traveled due south, you'll hit land at Cupsogue Beach County Park. Although

it boasts a beautiful, sandy beach and more than 1 mile of ocean shoreline, Cupsogue may be most famous as a wintering ground for gray and harbor seals. Walk its bayside beach or paddle nearby during the winter, and you'll probably be lucky enough to observe more than a few of these marine mammals swimming and frolicking in the water or sunning themselves on an exposed sandbar just off the beach. As with the nesting birds, give these creatures the space they deserve.

Now that you're floating just off the beach on the bay's southern shore, head west and you'll reach the inlet in about 0.5 mile. You'll know you're getting close when the beach to your left gets replaced with some stone riprap used to combat erosion. Depending on water conditions, you may be able to paddle straight out of the inlet and onto the Atlantic Ocean. Of course, wind, waves, and tides may all conspire to act against you and make

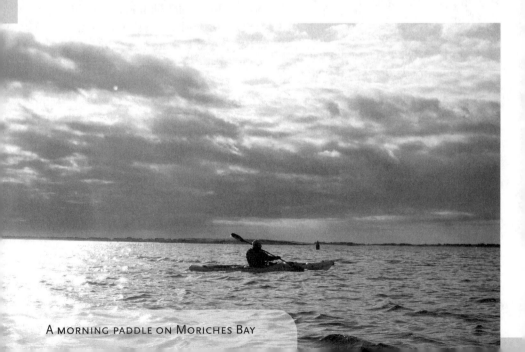

A MORNING PADDLE ON MORICHES BAY

this feat dangerous, if not impossible to accomplish. Rather than fight the elements in this case, a safer and likely more enjoyable option might be to avoid the inlet altogether by paddling east from Cupsogue Beach instead of west. This will give you an opportunity to explore the vast salt marsh that sits to the right of Cupsogue, and to check out the hundreds of beautiful beachfront homes built just beyond that.

Once you've had your fill of beach houses or played long enough in the Atlantic surf, simply turn your bow to the north and head back to the peninsula you started from. You should have a clear view of the Coast Guard station from most points in the bay, so the return trip will likely be an easy one.

◇ **SHUTTLE DIRECTIONS** To get to your put-in at the New York State boat ramp, take Sunrise Highway (NY 27) to Exit 59S. Get on the south service road and take it east 1.25 miles before turning right onto Railroad Avenue. Take Railroad Avenue south 1.6 miles until you reach Montauk Highway (NY 27A). Turn left onto Montauk Highway and travel 1.7 miles. Turn right onto Atlantic Avenue and take it south 0.8 mile. Keep an eye out for signs directing you to the Moriches Coast Guard Station.

- -

20 MT. SINAI HARBOR

◇ **OVERVIEW** Families looking for a quiet place to spend a day on the water, novice paddlers seeking a place to hone their skills, and experienced paddlers looking to pass a few hours in protected waters will all enjoy Mt. Sinai Harbor. Just east of Port Jefferson Harbor, it's small and quiet and great for paddling.

Since it was first settled, the town of Mt. Sinai has had more than its share of place-names. Native Americans called it *Nonowatuck,* or "Stream That Dries Up." After the English purchased the land from the Native Americans in 1664, they named it Old Mans, after an elderly fellow named Major Gotherson who lived in the area. In 1840 that name was deemed unseemly and changed yet again, this time for good. The story goes that the town postmaster opened his Bible and pointed a knitting needle at a random page. He chose the name closest to the needle.

Regardless of what you call it, Mt. Sinai offers much to see and do. Sunbathe on the town beach, have a go at fishing off the pier, or tie up your boat at Ralph's Fishing Station and get a grilled cheese at the snack bar. Of course, don't forget the main reason you came here—to paddle!

Because the harbor is small, you can explore every inch of it by kayak. Boat-watch while paddling through the mooring fields of the northern harbor, or bird-watch in the southern section. Land your boat on a small, sandy spit of land in the center of the harbor and have lunch. Or explore the narrow creeks near the western shore. Any or all of these options will yield an enjoyable day.

You'll find a few places to launch a kayak along the harbor's shoreline. Brookhaven Town residents may enter Cedar Beach Town Park and park near the fishing pier at the end of Harbor Beach Road. There is also a small dirt turnoff on Harbor Reach Road, about 0.5 mile east of Cedar Beach, from which boats can be launched. The best spot to put in, though, is Satterly Landing, on the harbor's southern shore. It's open to everyone during daylight hours and is free of charge.

USGS Quadrangles
PORT JEFFERSON (NY)

20 **DESCRIPTION** Because of its small size, you can see almost all of the harbor when launching from Satterly Landing. The moored and docked boats are visible to the north, just beyond the large marsh islands in the harbor's center. More marshland spreads out the east, and some high, tree-lined bluffs are obvious to the west. One of my favorite spots is a hidden treasure: a small creek in the harbor's southwest corner, less than a mile west of Satterly Landing.

You'll pass a few creeks and small breaks in the vast spartina marsh as you head west along the south shore. High water levels can make these fun places to explore. In addition, there's a small, sandy beach a little less than 0.5 mile from Satterly Landing; if need be, you can stop and rest here before you head any farther. Paddling just a few hundred feet farther, however, will bring you into a fairly large cove in the back harbor, overlooked by some large condos and houses.

Around the Harbor

Level	2A
Distance	4 miles around
Time	2 hours
Navigable months	Year-round
Hazards	Boat traffic on northern side
Portages	None
Rescue access	Limited
Tidal conditions	4 hours before or after high tide
Scenery	B+

Skirting the land's edge upon entering the cove will bring you to the small creek I mentioned a few sentences earlier. While not lengthy by any means, it's incredibly secluded, quiet, and beautiful. Spartina grasses line the waterways, and large beech trees hang overhead. Barely any sunlight penetrates to the water, making the old and abandoned wooden ship at the creek's dead end all the more fascinating to observe.

Heading north from the entrance to the creek will bring you to another quiet portion of Mt. Sinai's waters. Stay silent as you wind your way through the watery mazes here, and you may sneak up on one of the harbor's resident birds, the yellow-crowned

GPS COORDINATES

Put-in/take-out
N40° 57.206' W73° 01.817'
Tide station
Mt. Sinai Harbor, NY
N40° 57.798' W73° 02.399'

Mt. Sinai Harbor: Around the Harbor

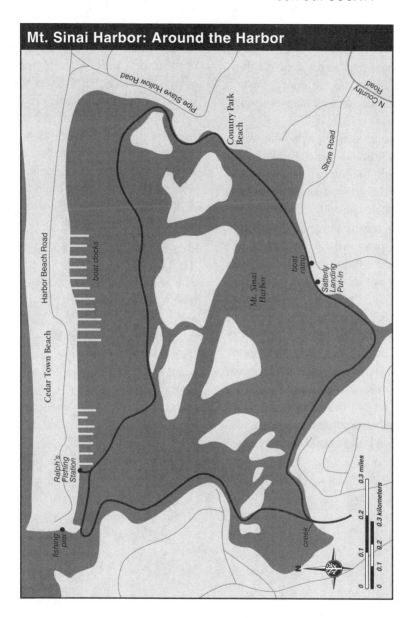

Pipe Stave Hollow Road

Country Park Beach

N County Road

Shore Road

Harbor Beach Road

boat docks

Cedar Town Beach

boat ramp

Satterly Landing Put-In

Mt. Sinai Harbor

Ralph's Fishing Station

fishing pier

creek

0.3 miles

0.2

0.3 kilometers

0.2

0.1

0.1

0

0

N

night heron. This beautiful bird stands almost 2 feet tall, with a long neck and bright white cheek feathers on its black face. You may even be lucky enough to see it catch its prey: these birds are the only species of heron that feeds on crustaceans.

Continuing north will bring you to the harbor's inlet after just 0.5 mile of paddling. With a sharp bend along its route, a narrow width between its breakwaters, a fair amount of boat traffic, and a long fishing pier on its eastern side, this inlet is difficult to navigate by kayak. The safest route for heading out into Long Island Sound is to hug the western breakwater, staying out of both boaters' and anglers' ways.

If you aren't seeking more-open waters, though, turn east and paddle along the harbor's northern side. Note the red and green buoys marking the boat channel, and stay well outside their borders.

Instead of dealing with boat traffic, you may find it easier to head slightly south from the inlet and follow the edges of the grassy islands in the center of the harbor. As with the harbor's other marshes, these islands are made up of spartina, or salt-marsh cordgrass. This grass thrives there, getting inundated with salt water twice a day. Just above the high-tide line lives another type of spartina, called salt-meadow cordgrass. Unlike its cousin, this type of grass is ill-suited for frequent drowning, although it does appreciate a little salt-water bath now and again.

You can paddle the length of these islands (about 0.75 mile) or wind your way through the mazes of channels

between them. Either way, the scenery is delightful. The far eastern portion of the harbor widens a bit as the grass islands in the center give way to open water. This shoreline is also more developed, with numerous houses lining the waterfront. A small beach associated with another county park is about halfway down the eastern shore, complete with some short hiking trails and good picnic spots. From there, Satterly Landing is only 0.5 mile away to the west.

◇ **SHUTTLE DIRECTIONS** To get to the Satterly Landing put-in, take I-495 (the Long Island Expressway) to Exit 63N (CR 83). Take CR 83 north 8 miles and turn right onto NY 25A. After 0.4 mile, turn left onto Echo Avenue, then left again onto Pipe Stave Hollow Road. After 1 mile, turn left again onto North Country Road. After 0.25 mile, turn right onto Shore Road. Look for Satterly Landing on the left side of the road, 0.75 mile distant.

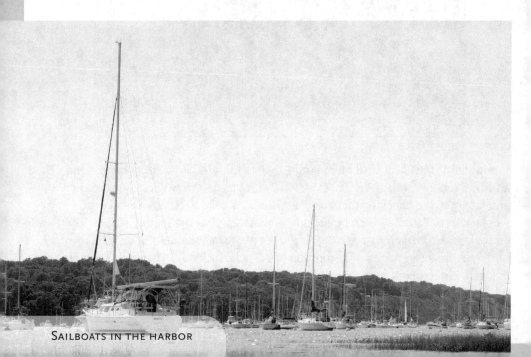

SAILBOATS IN THE HARBOR

21 NAPEAGUE HARBOR

✧ **OVERVIEW** Napeague Harbor lies on the South Fork of Long Island, about as far east as one can get (only the town of Montauk resides beyond). When you see the harbor, it's easy to see why the Montaukett people who once inhabited the area named it "Land Overflowed by the Sea." True to form, it's only about 1.5 miles long, 1 mile wide, and rarely more than a few feet deep. What Napeague Harbor lacks in size, however, it makes up for in history, nature, and ideal weather.

During the 17th century, the area around the harbor was a source of wood for New York City and Connecticut. Throughout the 18th and 19th centuries, the harbor became the site of no less than ten fish factories that processed menhaden for oil. Next came fish farming, a radio tower brought from Pearl Harbor after the infamous attack, an oddly appealing barge that houses an art school, and finally the draw of the Hamptons summer crowds. In short, the harbor's waters have seen a lot.

Napeague Harbor also has some amazing natural beauty to go along with its storied past. Indeed, the area is perhaps best known as the site of the remarkable "Walking Dunes." These huge mounds of sand, some reaching upwards of 75 feet, appear to be walking as they are blown to the southeast 3–4 feet a year. As the dunes move, they pass over sections of forest, leaving only treetops exposed at their peaks and stumps of dead trees at their bases. The dunes also surround a small freshwater bog that grows a crop of cranberries each fall. The dunes, the treetops and stumps, and the cranberry bog are all accessible from a short hiking trail that winds its way through the area.

The same prevailing winds that cause the dunes here to "walk" have also created another unique situation: the perfect windsurfing spot. Windsurfers, and more recently kiteboarders, now come to Napeague to take advantage of these winds, the harbor's limited boat traffic, and its shallow waters. In fact, Napeague Harbor has become one of the premier sailing locations on the East Coast. It is these same conditions (minus the wind, of course) that also make it an ideal paddling location.

A few put-ins exist along the harbor's shores, although most require an East Hampton town permit. My favorite put-in, at the Walking Dunes trailhead, is free and available to anyone. It's just a short drive down a dead-end road, has ample parking for more than a few cars, and provides easy access to the water. In fact, you can see most of the harbor from the beach there and choose in which direction to proceed. North? South? West? It's hard to decide.

USGS Quadrangles
GARDINERS ISLAND EAST (NY), NAPEAGUE BEACH (NY)

21 DESCRIPTION After you launch from the beach at the Walking Dunes trailhead, heading north will bring

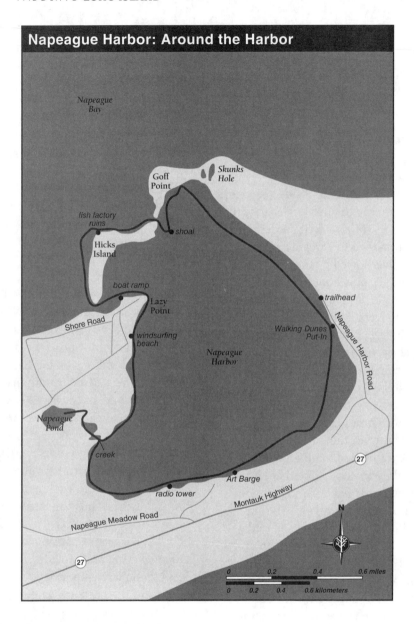

Napeague Harbor: Around the Harbor

you to another trail on the beach, just a few hundred feet away. Kayakers can easily pull up their craft onto the beach and follow the trail deep into the center of the amazing walking dunes. Those already committed to a day on the water can continue north along Napeague's shoreline and view some of these amazing natural features from their boats. Even when viewed from the seat of a kayak, the color of the sand on the beach should be quite hard to miss. Its striking rust hue is the result of a chemical reaction between the large amounts of iron in the surrounding seawater and the oxygen in the air. When exposed to the air, the iron oxidizes and forms actual rust.

Not much in the way of vegetation grows along the rusty beaches on this side of the harbor. A few small tufts of beach grass and some small salt-loving shrubs have taken root in the ever-shifting sands in some places, although the winds and salt air have surely kept their growth limited.

The northernmost portion of Napeague, Goff Point, comes just 1 mile from the put-in. Boats can also be easily landed here, although portions of the beach may be closed due to nesting bird colonies. Every spring, endangered piping plovers and least terns come here to try their luck at nesting on a fairly exposed piece of land. These birds have enough trouble doing so with scavengers like foxes and raccoons constantly on the prowl, and they definitely don't need people to make things tougher. Luckily for them, the New York State Department of Environmental Conservation closes off sections of nesting habitat from foot and vehicular traffic at the start of each nesting season. If you happen to paddle here during spring or summer and find certain areas of beach closed, do the plovers and terns a favor and keep clear.

If the beaches here are open, however, they're a great starting point for crossing Goff Point and spending some time on Napeague Bay and Block Island Sound. A short walk to a shallow pond known as Skunk's Hole may also be in order. In the northeasternmost corner of the harbor, the pond makes for a quick and convenient side trip that, thankfully, involves no skunks. From Skunk's Hole, the harbor's inlet

Around the Harbor

Level	2A
Distance	6 miles around
Time	3 hours
Navigable months	Year-round
Hazards	Winds
Portages	None
Rescue access	Limited
Tidal conditions	3 hours before or after high tide
Scenery	A

sits just a few hundred feet to the southwest, providing boat access to the sound. Any paddler heading this way should look out for a fairly large shoal that lies southeast of the inlet—at low tides, it can be enough to ruin a day.

Napeague Harbor's entrance would be a lot wider were it not for an island lying right in the middle of it. Called Hicks Island, this piece of land was created mainly from sand dredged from the area. The island was home to a fish factory in the late 1800s, the remnants of which can still be found on the island's northern side, and is now designated as a bird sanctuary. Hicks Island is a popular place to observe migrating and wintering waterfowl like mergansers and buffleheads, but it also boasts a large population

GPS Coordinates

Put-in/take-out
N41° 00.645' W72° 02.263'
Tide station
Promised Land, Napeague Bay, NY
N40° 59.899' W72° 04.902'

of spring and summer shorebirds. In fact, in just a short amount of time I was able to spot common terns, American oystercatchers, ruddy turnstones, swallows, willets, dunlins, black-bellied plovers, and a great blue heron the last time I paddled here.

Hicks Island is only about 0.5 mile long from top to bottom, so paddling around it is a breeze. A rocky piece of land called Lazy Point sticks out just south of the island; many of the area's fishermen launch their boats from here. Kayakers may launch from here as well, but only those with East Hampton town permits. Luckily, 0.3 mile from Lazy Point is a small beach popular among the local windsurfing crowd. Launching access is open to all, although the parking is a bit tricky. Your best bet is to drop off your boat and gear at the water's edge but park down the road a bit, beyond the NO PARKING signs.

Once you round Lazy Point and paddle past the windsurfers, nothing but spartina grass, a few pine trees, and some short stretches of sand will be in your line of sight. A handful of small cottages sit on the water's edge about 0.5 mile south of Lazy Point, but they disappear just before a small creek empties into the harbor to the right (west). Follow this creek when water levels are high enough, and you'll soon enter Napeague Pond. The pond, surrounded on all sides by an extensive salt marsh, is a likely place to spy a red-tailed hawk or osprey flying above. Even if you don't see any birds, just being in such a secluded location should be enough to make the side trip worthwhile.

Two additional creeks appear just a bit south of the first, both winding their way into the vast salt marsh in this corner of the harbor. Both are navigable, although barely, and should only be explored during periods of high tides, unless of course you desire a good dosing of mud. Following the harbor's shore to the east brings the large Mackay Radio Tower into view, with the locally famous "Art Barge" a bit farther in the distance. Once part of a pair that received and transmitted important messages from ships at sea, the sole standing radio tower now serves only a limited function broadcasting police communications. The aptly named Art Barge, however, is the site of many happenings, from classes to shows to a full gallery. Once seaworthy, the vessel now sits high and dry, an iconic landmark on the harbor.

A bit of road noise can be heard along this stretch of shoreline, as Montauk Highway comes into view to the south. Paddle a bit farther and, as if taking their cue from the road, houses appear once again. These quaint waterfront homes only add to Napeague Harbor's charm, though. Pass the northernmost house, and the Walking Dunes trailhead is just 0.25 mile away.

✧ **SHUTTLE DIRECTIONS** To get to the put-in at the Walking Dunes trailhead, take NY 27 (Montauk Highway) east through the town of Amagansett or west from Montauk. Turn north onto Napeague Harbor Road (between the Napeague Tennis Club and Cyril's Fish House) and continue 0.7 mile. The road will dead-end at the trailhead. Look for the put-in on the left.

22 NISSEQUOGUE RIVER

✧ **OVERVIEW** The Nissequogue is Long Island's third-longest river, flowing for 8 miles from its source in the center of the island to its mouth at Long Island Sound. Roughly 6 miles of navigable river take paddlers through many different habitats, including freshwater ponds, river tributaries, freshwater wetlands, brackish waters, and marine estuaries. Thankfully, the importance of protecting these wonderful natural resources was realized in 1982, when portions of the Nissequogue were added to the Wild, Scenic, and Recreational Rivers system.

Although parts of the river have been developed, its beauty has not been tarnished. Red maple, tulip, and locust trees still dominate the banks of the Nissequogue's upper portion, while spartina grasses and phragmites characterize the marshes of the lower river. Numerous species of birds, reptiles, and other animals also call the river home. Expect to see Canada geese, mute swans, and mallard ducks swimming along the water's surface, with snapping turtles and many species of crabs cruising below. Muskrats are very common along the river's muddy banks; terns, ospreys, and red-winged blackbirds fill the sky. The Nissequogue's clean water, combined with its gravel riverbed, makes it a great place for fishing. The river is naturally home to brown trout, bluefish, and

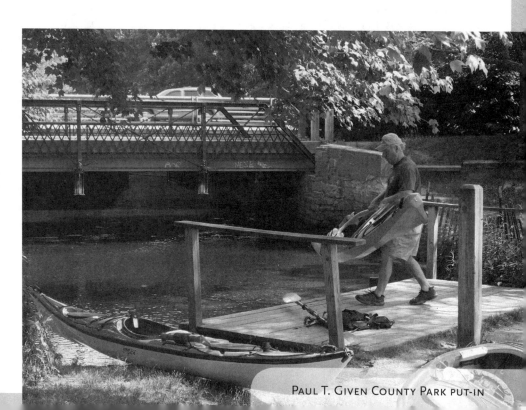

PAUL T. GIVEN COUNTY PARK PUT-IN

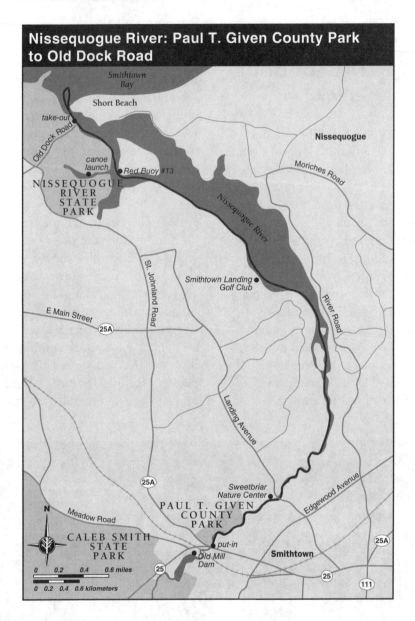

Nissequogue River: Paul T. Given County Park to Old Dock Road

striped bass and is stocked weekly during the spring and summer with rainbow and brook trout as well.

Because the Nissequogue is a tidal river, it can be run upstream or down, depending on the tides. The last 4 hours of a rising tide are perfect for a trip south, while the first 4 hours of a falling tide are great for a paddle north. Paddling during low tide is not recommended, though. (*Nissequogue* is a Native American word meaning "clay banks"—a fitting description of the river at low tide.)

USGS Quadrangles SAINT JAMES (NY), CENTRAL ISLIP (NY)

22 **DESCRIPTION** When beginning your trip from the Smithtown put-in, head south after entering the water and you will quickly reach a fork in the river. Taking either branch will allow you to explore the small dam and pond found there. The dam, built in the early 1800s, was used to power the local gristmill, remnants of which still stand along the riverbanks. After exploring this small section of river, turn around and head north, paddling under the concrete overpass for NY 25A. The road does add a lot of noise to the river, but that noise soon fades, leaving you with only the sounds of wildlife.

As you continue north along the very narrow lower Nissequogue, the shoreline changes from tree-lined to being bordered by phragmites. This invasive plant from Europe, identifiable by its tall and slender stalks and brownish-purple featherlike flowers at its tip, has taken over many an ecosystem on Long Island, and the Nissequogue is no exception. Although it is beautiful to look at, phragmites poses a serious threat to indigenous plant life, often outcompeting it for the resources necessary to grow and thrive. The plant can tolerate a wide range of salinity levels and is resistant to levels of pollution that would normally harm other species. As if these superhero-like powers weren't enough, phragmites can reproduce via underground stems known as rhizomes. This adaptation makes it extremely hardy and difficult to eradicate—cutting one stalk down does little to harm the main plant.

Wherever there are breaks in the phragmites, though, you can see the

Paul T. Given County Park to Old Dock Road

Level	1A
Distance	5.9 miles one-way
Time	3 hours
Navigable months	Year-round
Hazards	Boat traffic near northern end
Portages	None
Rescue access	Easy
Tidal conditions	4 hours before or after high tide
Scenery	A

river's shores. You'll notice that the majority of the eastern bank is lined with private homes, while most of the western bank is undeveloped. In fact, a section of this bank borders Sweetbriar Nature Center, a 54-acre park containing nature exhibits, a butterfly house, rehabilitated wildlife, and miles of hiking trails. Paddle down the small creek shown on the map, and you'll be able to land your boat and hike on the nature center's trails. You may also get out of your boat a bit farther north on the east side of the river at Landing Avenue Park. There is a playground there, as well as picnic tables and another short hiking trail to check out.

GPS Coordinates

Put-in
N40° 51.471' W73° 12.657'
Take-out
N40° 54.317' W73° 13.890'
Tide station
Nissequogue River Entrance, NY
N40° 54.000' W73° 13.998'

The Nissequogue twists and turns through more large swaths of phragmites as it winds its way downstream from Landing Avenue. It's never more than a few dozen feet wide in this section, giving paddlers plenty of opportunities to spy snapping turtles basking on the mud banks, red-winged blackbirds calling from the tops of the reeds, or dragonflies buzzing just above the water's surface. Much of the same continues for the next mile or so, until you come to an old wooden bridge on the right-hand (east) side of the river. Beyond this bridge, you should start to notice a few changes on the river. On shore, the cattails and phragmites of freshwater wetlands give way to the cordgrasses of salt marshes. Likewise, the ducks and swans of the lower river are replaced by the gulls, herons, and egrets of the marsh.

As the river widens, 1 mile after you pass the wooden bridge, a vast maze of large and small marsh-grass islands spreads across the river. Navigable only during high tides, this section of river can provide a unique and enjoyable way to get up close and personal with much of the wildlife found here. Great egrets will surely be seen wading through the shallows hunting for fish, just as great blue herons will hide until the last possible minute before taking flight with a cacophony of squawks in protest. Terns can often be seen flitting about overhead along this stretch of river, while small fish use its geography for protection under water. But while the wildlife here is usually unlimited, the water is not: you don't want to get caught in the grassy maze when the tide runs out, or you'll risk losing your shoes as you drag your boat through the deep, dark salt-marsh mud.

Beyond this large marsh, as the river bends to the north, the Smithtown Landing Golf Club should come into view. A small beach on the western bank, after the large wooden bulkhead, is a great place to take a break. You can land there and follow the trail to the country club for restrooms and water, or you can just sit on the beach, eat a snack, and relax a bit.

The river turns west after the golf club, where the old Kings Park Psychiatric Hospital looms over the horizon. The hospital was open for more than 100 years, and it sure looks it. Once a warehouse for the mentally ill, the hospital is rumored today to be haunted by the spirits of its patients. Although much of the property is closed to the public, New York State has taken it over and developed portions of it into Nissequogue River State Park. If you want to head for the small boat docks on shore, look for Sand Creek, a small, navigable stream on the left, just after you pass red buoy #13. The Nissequogue River State Park canoe and kayak launch is at the creek's end. You may choose to end your trip there if you're not interested in continuing farther north to Long Island Sound.

If you're not yet ready to end your trip, however, continue heading downriver. Pass the Smithtown boat ramps, follow the river to its mouth, and enter the sound. Once there, you can paddle west along the beaches of Sunken Meadow State Park or head east along Short Beach. Or simply poke around a bit, then head back upriver to the town boat ramps or the state-park boat launch, land your boat, and end your journey.

✧ **SHUTTLE DIRECTIONS** To get to the put-in in Smithtown, take I-495 (the Long Island Expressway to Exit 55N (Old Willets Path). Old Willets Path will take you 3 miles north to NY 25 (the Jericho Turnpike). Turn right onto NY 25. After 1.5 miles you will see the famous Smithtown Bull statue. Across from this statue, on your right,

is Paul T. Given County Park. You can park anywhere in the dirt lot by the boat launch.

To get to the take-out in Kings Park, turn left after leaving Paul T. Given County Park and bear right onto NY 25A (St. Johnland Road) just before the Smithtown Bull statue. Continue north 4 miles before turning right onto Old Dock Road. The take-out is at the end of Old Dock Road.

23 NORTHPORT HARBOR

✧ **OVERVIEW** Along Long Island's North Shore, at the eastern edge of what was once considered its "Gold Coast," lies bucolic Northport Harbor. An obvious focal point of the area, the harbor lies at the end of Northport Village's picturesque Main Street, where locals and visitors alike can sit and gaze upon its beautiful waters and stunning scenery. Also quite popular with the boating crowd, it's often filled to what looks like capacity with moored boats, although it still somehow manages to maintain its old-world charm.

Like most places on Long Island, Northport was first inhabited by the Native Americans, in this case the

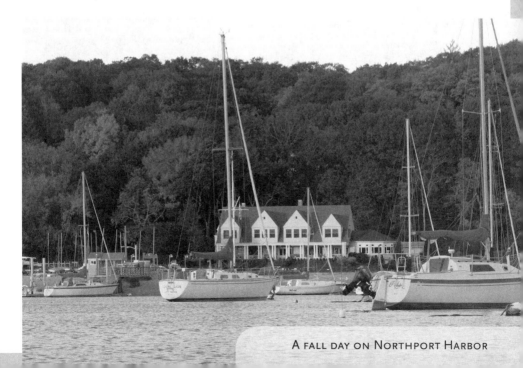

A FALL DAY ON NORTHPORT HARBOR

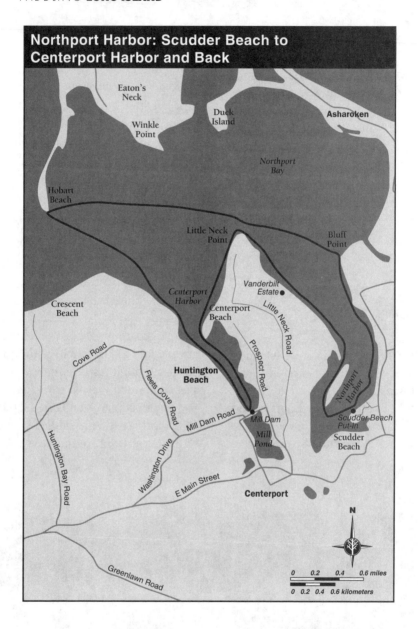

Northport Harbor: Scudder Beach to Centerport Harbor and Back

Eaton's Neck

Duck Island

Asharoken

Winkle Point

Northport Bay

Hobart Beach

Little Neck Point

Bluff Point

Vanderbilt Estate

Centerport Harbor

Crescent Beach

Centerport Beach

Little Neck Road

Cove Road

Prospect Road

Northport Harbor

Huntington Beach

Fleets Cove Road

Mill Dam Road

Mill Dam

Scudder Beach Put-In

Huntington Bay Road

Washington Drive

Mill Pond

Scudder Beach

E Main Street

Centerport

N

Greenlawn Road

0   0.2   0.4   0.6 miles

0   0.2   0.4   0.6 kilometers

Matinecocks, who were easily able to subsist on whatever they could harvest from the water and its surrounding lands. So deep was their appreciation of the harbor that they chose the place-name *Opcathontyche,* or "Wading-Place Creek." Even the Europeans who eventually purchased the land and harbor from the Matinecocks described it as having "good fishing, fine meadow-lands, and mostly level ground suitable for farms and cattle."

Although they did appreciate the potential their newly purchased land held, the new owners mainly used it mainly as grounds for grazing cattle. In fact, they quickly renamed the area Great Cow Harbor, after the area's most populous species. Indeed, the number of Northport residents remained quite low for many, many years, easily outnumbered by their livestock. It was not until the 19th century and the growth of the shipbuilding industry that this began to change.

Like many of the harbors around it, Northport took to shipbuilding with ease, making it the village's primary source of income by the end of the 1830s. Business was so good, in fact, that the village's name was officially changed to Northport in 1837 to reflect its maritime prosperity. Of course, the shipbuilding era eventually did come to a close, although Northport was able to survive its collapse with the help of a newly constructed Long Island Rail Road station and a successful downtown business district. Thankfully, it was also able to maintain its close ties to the water and remain a welcome harbor to all.

While Northport is truly a boaters' harbor, it definitely has a place for kayakers as well. Look to the very convenient boat ramp at Scudder Beach or the dock at Glacier Bay Sports if you want to come and explore its waters for yourself. Both put-ins are at the south end of the harbor.

USGS Quadrangles Northport (NY), Lloyd Harbor (NY)

23 **DESCRIPTION** Northport Harbor's popularity among the boating crowd will become immediately obvious once you launch from Scudder Beach. Although the scene directly in front of you appears wild and pristine

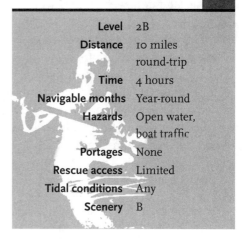

Scudder Beach to Centerport Harbor and Back

Level	2B
Distance	10 miles round-trip
Time	4 hours
Navigable months	Year-round
Hazards	Open water, boat traffic
Portages	None
Rescue access	Limited
Tidal conditions	Any
Scenery	B

(the small island is a bird sanctuary), it will seem as if the rest of the harbor is completely filled with boats. Indeed, an amazing number of moorings stretch along the harbor's length, and numerous docks line its shores. Remember, though: you're paddling a kayak. You don't need much room to navigate, nor do you need much water under your hull to progress forward. Simply paddle along the shore, between it and the edges of the mooring field, and you'll be safe and happy. Besides, the shores of Northport are where you'll find the most interesting things to look at.

Look to your right as you head north on the harbor, and you'll catch some good views of the houses built

GPS COORDINATES

Put-in/take-out
N40° 53.611' W73° 21.432'
Tide station
Northport Bay, NY
N40° 54.000' W73° 21.000'

atop the steeply sloped shoreline. A small marina will break up the view 0.4 mile later, followed almost immediately by a great view up Northport's Main Street. Seeing the town from such a vantage point is a treat that few on shore can really appreciate. Take a picture, enjoy the view, and then continue on, for there is more to see.

Once past Main Street and the town docks, you'll notice the harbor curving a bit to the west. The waterfront homes will once again dominate the shoreline, only to be interrupted by

a large yacht club 0.6 mile later. Its docks are home to some large and impressive boats, but they also mark a point where the general feel of the harbor changes. Take a look around as you sit in your kayak offshore of the yacht club, and you'll be able to feel this for yourself. You're only 0.25 mile away from the harbor's mouth at this point, floating on the boundary between the protected waters of Northport Harbor and those of the more exposed Northport Bay. At its widest stretch, the bay has a 3-mile fetch that can kick up

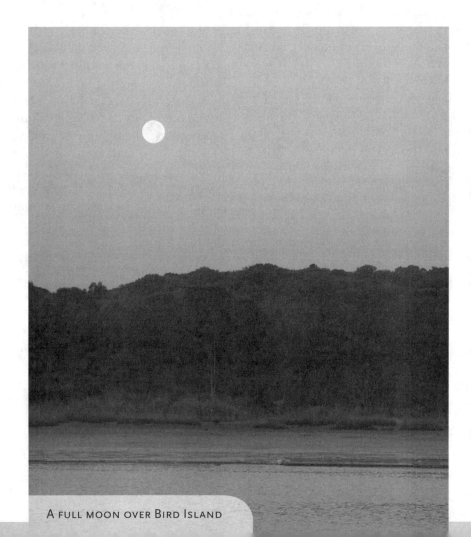

A FULL MOON OVER BIRD ISLAND

some pretty hefty waves whenever a decent wind (especially one from the west) is blowing.

Should you find yourself on Northport Harbor under such conditions, you may do well to remain within the relative safety of its confines. However, if the water is calm and Northport Bay looks inviting, you should definitely continue your paddle. A popular route from Northport Harbor is to continue paddling along the eastern shore and round the harbor's last point of land on this side, called Bluff Point. From there, unfortunately, views of the four smokestacks of Northport's power plant are unavoidable. Follow the shoreline to the north of the stacks, though, and you'll see a more welcoming sight: the causeway leading to Eatons Neck and tiny Duck Island Harbor. The harbor can be an amazing place to paddle should you choose this option. Likewise, the south shore of Eatons Neck can be a kayaker's paradise. In fact, if you turn your bow to the west upon leaving Northport Harbor instead of following the causeway, you'll come to a part of Eatons Neck that boasts one of the prettiest views along this entire stretch of water: the southern tip of Hobart Beach.

Getting to this part of Hobart Beach requires a 2.5-mile crossing over open water from Northport's Bluff Point, but the effort is quite worth it. Once you reach the tip of this sandy spit and are standing among its low-growing brush, you'll be treated to a 360-degree view of both Northport and Huntington bays, as well as Long Island Sound. The tip is also well situated for beginning a paddle to Huntington or

Lloyd Harbor or north around Eatons Neck, though Centerport Harbor is the usual destination.

Centerport's entrance is just 1.5 miles southeast of Hobart Beach, nestled between two public beaches that constrict the opening to just a few hundred feet wide. While one must be a town resident to park a car in the lot of either beach, paddlers can definitely land in both spots (outside of the marked swimming areas, of course) to stretch their legs, use the bathrooms, and have a quick bite or two to eat. After the crossing from Hobart Beach, this may be just what you're looking for.

Once you've passed through the opening into the harbor, you'll notice that it isn't very big at all. It runs only 0.6 mile to the southeast before it reaches the dam at Mill Dam Road. Paddle down its waters and you'll find many boats floating at their moorings, dozens of houses built right on the water's edge, and an amazing 22-foot-tall metal sculpture of a great blue heron sitting in the middle of a park in the harbor's southwest corner. As tall as it is, this bird is easily visible from most parts of the southern harbor, though you may want to take a closer look. If so, your only option is to paddle through the dam's opening in the center of Mill Dam Road. Of course, you can only do this during high tide; otherwise, the water pouring out of Mill Pond will make it impossible.

Given the names "Mill Dam Road" and "Mill Pond," it's easy to guess at what history this part of the harbor keeps. Sure enough, it was once the site of a tidal mill constructed in 1674. The original mill was replaced a century later by a gristmill, complete with a bridge that spanned the harbor from west to east. The second mill operated for almost a century and a half, until it was decommissioned and torn down. Unfortunately, most of its legacy has been lost, save for a millstone that was unearthed during construction of the new bridge and some wooden beams that were salvaged and used by William Vanderbilt in his nearby mansion. Still, it's always exciting to paddle through a bit of history.

As you turn your kayak to the north once again, stay close to the east side of the harbor and you'll encounter a large concrete wall painted with the name CAMP ALVERNIA. Built in 1888, Alvernia was the first Catholic summer camp in the country and was open only to boys. The camp is still run by the Franciscan Brothers of Brooklyn, making it the oldest continuously running Catholic camp in the United States, although it is now open to both boys and girls.

Head past the camp's property and you'll reach the harbor's entrance in 0.5 mile. You'll have to skirt around the sandbar that stretches out to the south from Centerport Beach on the right, but once around it you'll be back on the waters of Northport Bay. Follow the shore for the next mile, and you'll round Little Neck Point. Originally called Sills Point after Phineas Sills, one of the harbor's early settlers, Little Neck Point marks the western entrance to Northport Harbor.

Now that you're paddling back in Northport Harbor, pay attention as you continue down its western shore and you should find the Vanderbilt estate.

Although most of the railroad tycoon's 43-acre property can't be seen from the water, portions of it are quite easy to spot. The main building, called Crows Nest, is visible from the center and eastern portions of the harbor, whereas its elaborate but run-down beach house is on the water's edge, 0.5 mile south of Little Neck Point. Paddle just 0.2 mile farther, and what may be the estate's most unusual edifice will come into view. This old and dilapidated concrete structure was once the hangar where the Vanderbilt family stored and launched their seaplanes. The obvious deterioration of both the beach house and the hangar has made them off-limits to visitors, so for your own safety, observe them only from the seat of your kayak.

Hug the western shore as you continue paddling south, and you'll notice it gradually curving to the west. If you follow this curve past the docks of the Centerport Yacht Club, you won't be able to miss the small island identified earlier as a bird sanctuary. The aptly named Bird Island was created with the spoils of dredging and was then left to its own devices, free to grow and develop unmolested. It has since become an excellent spot for finding many bird species including Canada geese, great and snowy egrets, willets, brants (in the winter), and gulls. Amazingly, I once counted almost two dozen great blue herons on the island's shore and in its trees. Although Scudder Beach sits on shore to the east of Bird Island, I highly recommend taking the long way around the island's 0.3-mile length. You never know what you'll see there.

✧ **SHUTTLE DIRECTIONS** To get to the put-in at Scudder Beach, take the Northern State Parkway to Exit 42N (Deer Park Avenue). Follow the exit to East Deer Park Road and head north 0.8 mile until you reach NY 25. Turn right onto NY 25 and take your first left onto Elwood Road. Continue north on Elwood Road for 4 miles and turn left onto NY 25A. Follow NY 25A 0.5 mile before turning right onto Woodbine Avenue. Head north on Woodbine Avenue and look for Beach Avenue on your left after 0.25 mile. Turn onto Beach Avenue and follow the signs for Scudder Beach.

24 NORTH SEA HARBOR

✧ **OVERVIEW** Small in size but big in history, North Sea Harbor is another paddling destination on the South Fork of Long Island that shouldn't be missed. It's on Southampton's northern shore, between Cow Neck and North Sea, in a spot that provides perfect access to Little Peconic Bay. In fact, its location is so good that it was the landing spot of New York's first English settlers back in 1640. Although these men and women established the area's first town, Old Towne, about 4 miles to the south, they still relied on the harbor as an important seaport and used it as a port of entry for many years to come.

Today, visitors to the harbor will notice that there is no evidence of the Europeans' presence on its waters except for a plaque commemorating the occasion of their landing on Conscience Point. The Southampton Historical Museum is charged with preserving this historically significant location.

Preservation of another kind has also taken place on the harbor, with the creation of the Conscience Point National Wildlife Refuge. Made possible by a land grant in the early 1970s, the refuge was established to help protect the area's vanishing marine-grassland ecosystem. It also provides a safe habitat for not only migratory and wintering waterfowl but many species of shorebirds. The refuge has proved invaluable in maintaining the ecological biodiversity of North Sea Harbor.

Unfortunately, with numerous private waterfront homes on North Sea's eastern shore and a wildlife refuge along the western one, access to the harbor is somewhat limited. There is a put-in that anyone can use, though, along North Sea Road on the harbor's southern end. Canoes or kayaks can be easily launched from its ramp, putting all of the harbor's history and natural beauty at your fingertips.

USGS Quadrangles
SOUTHAMPTON (NY)

24 **DESCRIPTION** After you launch on North Sea Harbor, you can paddle down a small creek that runs for about 0.5 mile to the south. The creek is narrow, however, and is lined with houses and boat docks. A much better choice is to head north from the put-in and

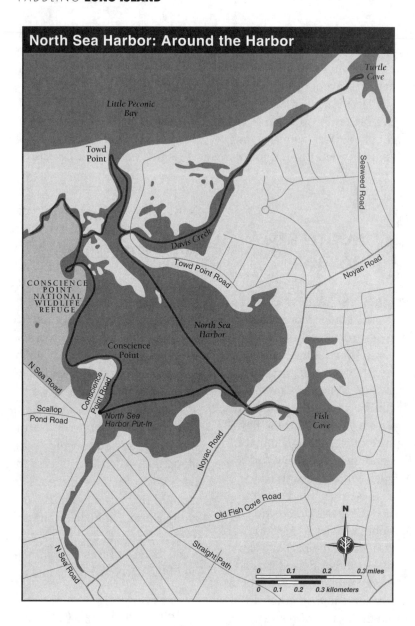

North Sea Harbor: Around the Harbor

check out the historically important Conscience Point.

This small piece of land jutting out into the harbor is where English colonists landed in 1640, subsequently creating the first European settlement in New York State, called Old Towne (known today as Southampton). Lore

has it that one of the original settlers, a woman, remarked upon landing, "For conscience sake, I am on dry land once more"—hence the point's name.

You can land a kayak at the tip of Conscience Point, where a small beach may be exposed during certain tide levels. After exploring this small area,

Around the Harbor

Level	2A
Distance	5.1 miles around
Time	2–3 hours
Navigable months	Year-round
Hazards	None
Portages	None
Rescue access	Easy
Tidal conditions	Any
Scenery	B+

most paddlers round the point and continue following the shoreline west, entering the Conscience Point National Wildlife Refuge. Part of this refuge, a small cove just south of Conscience Point, includes a shellfish-spawning area maintained by The Nature Conservancy. As an advocate for and protector of biodiversity, the conservancy has organized an immense shellfish-restoration project, including protected bodies of water across much of the East End of Long Island. Paddlers should feel welcome to explore this small cove but obviously should not do anything to harm the area.

Shellfish are not the only organisms protected along the western shore of North Sea Harbor. In fact, the wildlife refuge was set up largely to protect migratory birds and wintering waterfowl. Great blue herons, great and snowy egrets, red-winged blackbirds, common and least terns, and ospreys are all quite common here during the spring and summer. With fall and winter come the black ducks, buffleheads, and the occasional merganser or two. I even spied a group

of wild turkeys strutting along the shoreline the last time I paddled here. According to the refuge's website, it also protects some endangered maritime plants such as switchgrass, little bluestem, poverty grass, and hairgrass.

Continue north, following the harbor's western shore, and reach a small island just before the inlet. Skirt around the island's left side, and a small creek will appear on the mainland a bit to the north. It's a short side trip, but paddling down this creek will bring you into two consecutive pondlike bodies of water surrounded by spartina and lined with red maple, cedar, and cherry trees. Just a few hundred feet beyond the creek lies the harbor's inlet and Little Peconic Bay. Another side trip, this one a good deal longer, is possible once you're out on the bay. Robins Island sits roughly in the middle of the bay, just 2 miles distant. It's a worthy paddling destination in itself, although landing a boat anywhere on its beaches is prohibited.

Once you've explored Little Peconic Bay and the long, sandy beaches of Towd Point, you can paddle through another unique setting. Follow the eastern side of the inlet back into the harbor, and look for a bridge crossing a creek on the left side. Heading under this bridge will bring you to Davis Creek, a mile-long stretch of water that

GPS COORDINATES

Put-in/take-out
N40° 56.242' W72° 25.014'
Tide station
Shinnecock Canal, NY
N40° 54.000' W72° 30.000'

runs alongside a vast salt marsh to the north and dozens of houses to the south. The creek passes under eight wooden footbridges along the way, each built to give homeowners access to the bay beach to the north. The bridges also provide excellent nesting spots for barn swallows, scores of which can be seen resting underneath or flying above the wooden structures.

North Sea Harbor offers paddlers one more surprise, with 1.5 additional miles of shoreline to explore. Paddling out of Davis Creek and less than a mile across the harbor to the southeast will bring you to this small area, known as Fish Cove. Look for its entrance under the stone bridge, just right (east) of a small, sandy beach. The cove is somewhat small and lined with homes on all sides. When you're ready to end your trip, the boat ramp is just 0.5 mile due west from the same stone bridge that leads to Fish Cove.

⟡ **SHUTTLE DIRECTIONS** To get to the put-in on North Sea Road, take NY 27 into the town of Southampton. Turn left onto North Sea Road if coming from the west, right if coming from the east. Continue north 2.5 miles, at which time North Sea Road meets Noyack Road. Keep left here and follow North Sea Road for an additional 0.5 mile. Look for a dirt road and boat ramp on the right-hand side of the road.

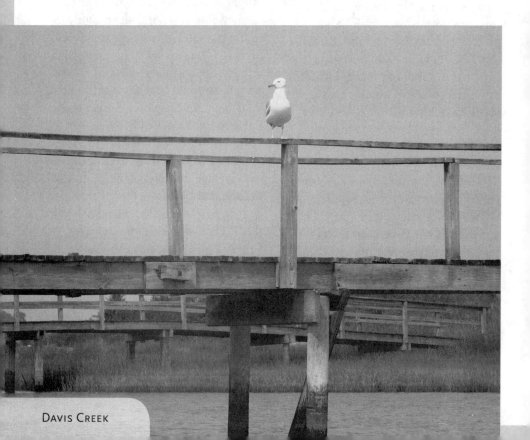

DAVIS CREEK

25 PECONIC RIVER

◇ **OVERVIEW** The Peconic is Long Island's longest river, flowing east 15 miles from underground springs near the center of the island to its mouth at Peconic Bay. On its way, the river passes through such diverse habitats as freshwater swamps and bogs, farmland, and oak forests. In addition, it flows through a portion of the Long Island Pine Barrens region that provides not only a critical habitat for a variety of wildlife but also clean, fresh drinking water for Long Island's residents.

The Peconic also passes through some historic areas where residents once farmed cranberries and forged iron. Cranberry farming was so successful on the Peconic that the area was once the third-largest cranberry producer in the nation. Likewise, the iron deposits in the Peconic's bogs were so vast that large anchors and metal hulls for Civil War–era ironclad ships were easily produced there.

These days the Peconic is most popular as a paddling destination. The iron forges and cranberry farms are gone, leaving a beautiful, scenic river in their place. The riverbanks are lined with red maples and willow trees, pitch-pine and oak trees tower overhead, and water willow and phragmites dominate the water's edge. Expect to see swans, wood ducks, cedar waxwings, ospreys, and kingfishers flying along the river's course, while muskrats, snapping turtles, bluegills, and largemouth bass swim in its waters.

Because of its scenery, calm water, numerous put-ins, and nearby canoe-rental facilities, the Peconic River can get very crowded, especially on

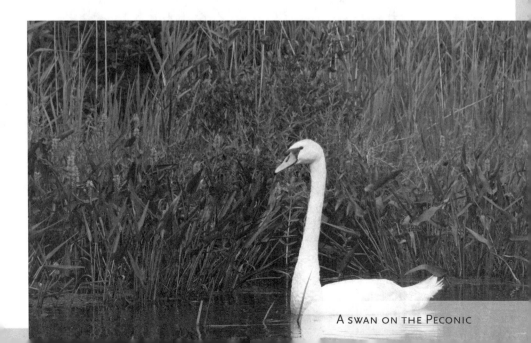

A SWAN ON THE PECONIC

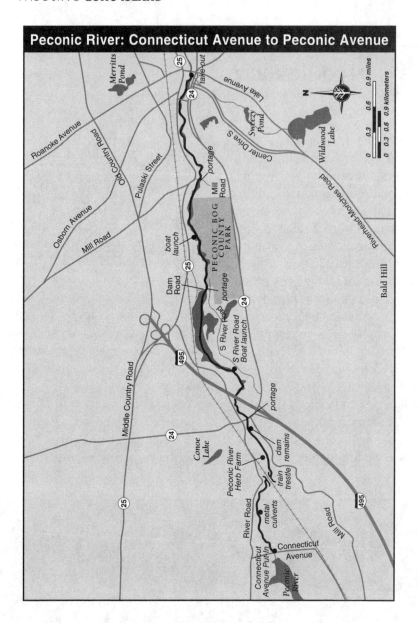

Peconic River: Connecticut Avenue to Peconic Avenue

summer weekends. Be ready to share the river with other canoeists and kayakers, as well as local fishermen. Whether done alone or with a group, though, paddling the Peconic River is an incredibly enjoyable adventure.

USGS Quadrangles WADING RIVER (NY), RIVERHEAD (NY)

25 **DESCRIPTION** Although there are numerous put-ins along the Peconic River, most paddlers begin their trip at Connecticut Avenue in Calverton, where the river is very narrow and shallow but also wild and scenic. During late spring and summer, it is usually enveloped with the fragrance of the plentiful wildflowers that grow on its banks. Expect to see (and smell) small stalks of sweet pepperbush and strands of purple swamp loosestrife curving down to the water in great abundance here.

Later in the year, this same stretch of river glows with the vibrant colors of autumn. Although they keep some of their signature color all year long, the red maples along the Peconic are particularly beautiful in October and early November. Add to them the striking reds of the tupelo trees and the bright yellows of the willows that share the dry ground, and it's easy to get lost in the beauty of the river.

After you've paddled 0.25 mile, the river opens up a bit, introducing you to one of the most insidious invasive plants inhabiting Long Island's aquatic ecosystems. Called phragmites, or common reed, it's easily identifiable by its tall, slender shape, with featherlike flowers in tufts on top. Phragmites is well adapted to life in aquatic ecosystems like the Peconic River and, as such, outcompetes local plants for space and nutrients. Unfortunately, it is also extremely difficult to eradicate, which causes even bigger problems for cattails and other indigenous species. Phragmites will be a constant companion from this point of the river on—a testament to its regrettable success.

After another 0.25 mile, four metal culverts that pass under an overgrown dirt path will come into view. While the opening farthest to the left is almost completely blocked off, the remaining three are free and clear. The easiest path lies through the culvert

Connecticut Avenue to Peconic Avenue

Level	1B
Distance	7.1 miles one-way
Time	3–4 hours
Navigable months	Year-round
Hazards	None
Portages	4
Rescue access	Easy
Tidal conditions	Spring-fed—not affected by tides
Scenery	B+–A

farthest to the right. A beautiful yet tiny purple flower named bittersweet nightshade thrives in the portion of the river immediately after the culverts. It grows as a vine and produces a flower with five purple petals and a bright-yellow stamen. Look at the plant, admire its beauty, and take a photo or two, but do no more than that: both the flower and its berries are poisonous if ingested.

As a safer (and tastier) alternative, stop and sample the crops at the Peconic River Herb Farm, less than 1 mile downstream of the metal culverts, on the left side of the river (631-369-0058; **prherbfarm.com**). Paddlers may make use of the farm's picnic tables and can purchase a wide variety of plants for home and garden. Even if you don't

GPS COORDINATES

Put-in
N40° 54.043' W72° 46.410'
Take-out
N40° 54.932' W72° 39.826'

care to eat or shop, you can still walk around and enjoy the scenery.

You may have noticed the remains of a large earthen dam crossing the river just before the herb farm. This dam, like the one that comes shortly after, was built by local cranberry farmers to flood the river and create the boglike conditions that are suitable for growing the delicious red fruit. When you consider how wide and shallow the river is in this section, it's obvious that the farmers knew what they were doing.

After passing through the first dam, enjoying a rest and a chance to shop at the herb farm, and continuing beyond the second earthen dam, keep heading east and weave your way through what is one of my favorite parts of the Peconic—marked by the striking white flowers of fragrant water lilies and the bulbous yellow flowers of yellow pond lilies. Few spots on Long Island support as large a number of these water lilies as on this section of the river.

The Peconic flows over another dam at Edwards Avenue, 0.5 mile after the old cranberry farm. This dam requires a portage, made easier by a set of wooden stairs and a boat ramp. Still, the water currents can be quite swift and unpredictable as the river flows under the road. Sure feet, arm strength, and a paddling partner's help can make a world of difference here.

The river narrows again once you've crossed Edwards Avenue. A half-mile later, it passes under Interstate 495 (Long Island Expressway), through two concrete culverts with low ceilings, and eventually flows into Peconic Lake. Local fishermen frequent the lake in search of bass, bluegill, sunfish and other freshwater species, plying the waters in small boats with electric motors. Thankfully, these will be the only motorboats you will see on the whole river. You'll reach the eastern shore of the lake after 1 mile, requiring a second portage. You will need to cross Forge Road, named after an iron forge that existed there 200 years ago, and slide your boat down the wooden ramp on the other side. The river takes on a different feel from this point on, as natural wetlands give way to developed tracts of land. You will paddle past numerous houses, businesses, and side roads as you continue your trip east. Thankfully, the remaining land is fairly wooded, with the usual red maples, oaks, and tupelo trees that one would expect to find in freshwater environments.

Your third portage occurs 1.5 miles past Forge Road. Most paddlers consider this portage the fun one because of the ice-cream stand and Mexican restaurant just a short walk away. Get your fill of burritos and ice-cream cones; then carry your boat across Mill Road and through the small dirt parking lot, and reenter the water on the other side. A concrete dam immediately after the portage will require you to get out of your boat one last time. You can carry your boat over the waterfall quite easily on the right-hand (south) side of the river.

The sights and sounds of civilization become more pronounced during your last mile of paddling on the Peconic. A few riverside businesses and houses soon appear, as does a large white-and-blue water tower emblazoned with the town's name. This section of the river ends at Grangebel Park. (Construction was started in the park during the spring of 2010 and has yet to be completed. Although installation of a canoe-and-kayak ramp in the park has been proposed, it has not been built as of this writing.) Look for your take-out at the beach of the Peconic Paddler canoe and kayak store, on the far-right-hand side of the park.

✧ **SHUTTLE DIRECTIONS** To get to your put-in on Connecticut Avenue, take I-495 (the Long Island Expressway) to Exit 71N (NY 24). Travel north on NY 24, taking the third left onto River Road. Head west on River Road 1.8 miles and you will reach Connecticut Avenue on your left. You will see the sign for the Peconic River put-in on the left, 0.3 mile down the road.

To get to your take-out at Peconic Paddler in Riverhead, take I-495 to Exit 72S (NY 25). Travel east on NY 25 toward the town of Riverhead. You will reach a traffic light at Peconic Avenue after 3.5 miles. Turn right there and you will see Peconic Paddler on the right-hand side of the road. You may pick up or drop off any boats and gear in front of the store, but you should park across the street in the public parking lot.

26 PORT JEFFERSON HARBOR

✧ **OVERVIEW** Imagine a place where ferries and sailboats, megayachts and rowboats, Jet Skis and kayaks can all get along. Port Jefferson Harbor is such a place. It sits on Long Island Sound, about halfway between New York City and Orient Point, with enough water inside its boundaries to provide room for everyone. The working boats stay to the west, recreational boats to the east, small sailboats to the south, weekend sailors to the north, and kayakers in between. Factor in beautiful beaches, rich history, and a quaint harbor-side town, and Port Jefferson's popularity is easy to figure out.

Like many places along Long Island, Port Jefferson was once inhabited by Native Americans—the Setalcotts, in this case. This group named the area *Sowassett,* or "Where Water Opens Out," probably referring to the marshy land that was frequently flooded by tides. Port Jefferson's first settler, John Roe, seemed to agree with the Setalcotts' description of the place: he named it Drowned Meadow after he arrived there in 1682. Many settlers soon followed in Roe's footsteps, developing the harbor and its surrounding lands into a bustling seaport.

Shipbuilding began on the harbor in the 1800s and became an extremely lucrative business. In fact, it was this industry that ultimately led to the harbor's name change. In 1836, locals decided that "Drowned Meadow" was not the best name for a town where ships were built. Port Jefferson was chosen as its new name, partly to thank the third President of the United States for helping fund flood-prevention efforts in the town.

Port Jefferson Harbor: Around the Harbor

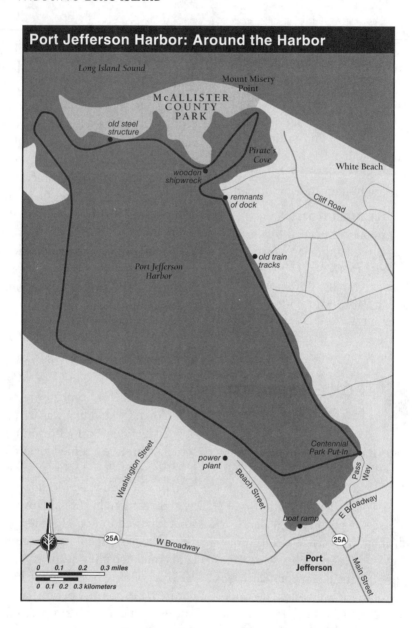

Long Island Sound

Mount Misery Point

McALLISTER COUNTY PARK

old steel structure

wooden shipwreck

Pirate's Cove

White Beach

remnants of dock

Cliff Road

Port Jefferson Harbor

old train tracks

power plant

Centennial Park Put-In

Washington Street

Beach Street

Pass Way

E Broadway

boat ramp

N

25A

W Broadway

25A

Main Street

Port Jefferson

0   0.1   0.2   0.3 miles

0   0.1   0.2   0.3 kilometers

The shipbuilding industry eventually left, but Port Jefferson's rich maritime history is still very much alive and visible. Today, dozens of historic homes overlook the harbor, tracks from an old shipway (building platform) are visible where an old shipyard stood, and even a dilapidated shipyard building was saved and converted into a beautiful village center.

A ferry terminal has helped solidify Port Jefferson's importance as a harbor, although the town would likely be able to survive based on its restaurants, ice-cream and souvenir shops, nightclubs, and hotels alone.

It truly is a tourist town, although locals love it as well. Owning a boat or kayak just makes it better. Most of the harbor's southern end is lined with docks and parking lots, though a quieter, paddler-friendly put-in lies on the eastern side of the harbor, in Port Jefferson's Centennial Park. The pluses: free parking (just a short walk from town), a sandy beach, and quiet water.

USGS Quadrangles
PORT JEFFERSON (NY)

26 **DESCRIPTION** In a harbor with as much boat traffic (including a large car ferry) as Port Jefferson's, it's best to paddle as far away from the boat channel as possible. Launching from the Centennial Park beach and hugging the eastern shore of the harbor lets you do just that. As luck would have it, this shore is also less developed, making it a pleasure to paddle.

Head straight off the beach, and the first things you'll paddle past are the small boats of the local sailing school. Come here on a windy day and you'll definitely enjoy watching kids learn the finer arts of seamanship. Beyond the junior sailboats, a large mooring field stretches to the northwest for more than a mile. Everything from small fishing boats and powerboats to sailboats and some larger yachts can be found here, making it a boat-watcher's dream come true. You could easily spend an hour or two winding your way among the many different boats on your way to the outer harbor.

For those not wishing to get up close and personal with larger

Around the Harbor

Level	2A
Distance	5.4 miles around
Time	3 hours
Navigable months	Year-round
Hazards	Boat traffic
Portages	None
Rescue access	Easy
Tidal conditions	Any
Scenery	A

watercraft, a fairly wide channel of water exists between the far right edge of the mooring field and the harbor's eastern shore. This quieter, more protected stretch of water gives you the chance to observe the narrow, rocky beach along the harbor's edge and peek at the few houses hidden among the tree-lined bluffs. A decent-sized dock juts into the harbor about 0.5 mile north of Centennial Park, with a few more coming up after that. They do little to mar the view, however, or make paddling difficult or unsafe.

More interesting to look at, though, are the remnants of the harbor's sand-and-gravel-mining operations, which were active during the late 19th and early 20th centuries. Visible are a portion of train track 1 mile from Centennial Park, an old wooden dock and

GPS COORDINATES

Put-in/take-out
N40° 57.054' W73° 04.028'
Tide station
Port Jefferson Harbor Entrance, NY
N40° 58.257' W73° 05.588'

concrete structure 0.2 mile beyond, some old wooden buildings across the boat channel on the far beach, even a partially buried ship's hull. While the decades-old ruins are amazing to look at, they can also be quite dangerous to paddle too close to. Admire them only from a safe distance.

When you reach the northeast-ernmost corner of the harbor, a fairly large cove becomes visible just before you cross over to the far beach. Known as Pirate's Cove, it owes its existence to the same mining opera-tions that left their ruins scattered about. Surrounded on three sides by large sand dunes, Pirate's Cove is an immensely popular place for boat-ers to moor and spend some time. In fact, on busy summer weekends,

it's almost possible to cross the cove without getting wet by walking across the boats floating there. I consider Pirate's Cove one of my top ten pretti-est places on Long Island, and I visit it as often as possible (except during its busiest times).

Just across the channel leading to Pirate's Cove sits a fairly large and undeveloped piece of land known as Mt. Misery Point. Now home to McAllister County Park, this area was once considered a barren waste-land. In fact, it was this desolation that earned the point its name: back in 1665, the Reverend Nathaniel Brewster landed there and exclaimed, "Oh, what a mountain of misery!" Many people disagree with the rev-erend's assessment, however, and

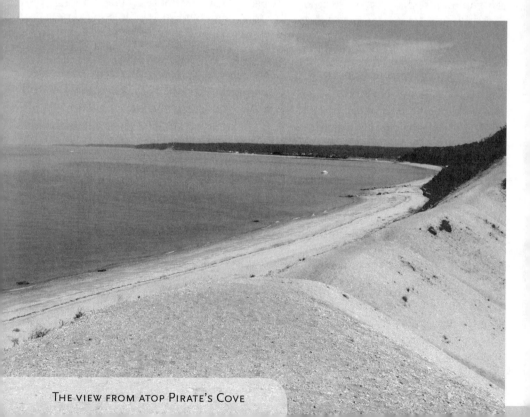

THE VIEW FROM ATOP PIRATE'S COVE

consider it a place of natural beauty. Regardless of your opinion, if you follow its shoreline to the west, you'll come to the harbor's inlet in 0.5 mile.

Great care should be taken when crossing this inlet. There is little room between the two breakwaters, the currents can move quite swiftly, there is usually boat traffic, and every so often a large ferry passes through. In short, the inlet can be a dangerous place to paddle, although crossing it provides access to the western side of the harbor.

If you choose to cross, you'll be paddling along another strip of land, Old Field Beach, separating the harbor from Long Island Sound. Like Pirate's Cove, it can be a busy place during the summer. Also like Pirate's Cove, it's a beautiful place and is worthy of a stop. After stretching your legs here, continue west and you can paddle into Setauket Harbor or Conscience Bay. Alternately, you can turn south and paddle the half-mile of water between Old Field Beach and Port Jefferson's western shore. This shore is more developed than its eastern counterpart, with houses, decks, and wooden stairs covering almost every available space. There is also a large industrial power plant on the water's edge, just 1 mile down the shoreline. It's hard to miss the plant's two red-and-white smokestacks, which can usually be seen for miles.

Obviously, paddling along the docks of a power plant requires a certain degree of caution and common sense. Most importantly, you should maintain a safe distance from the dock or any tankers or tugboats in the area.

You're not home free, though, once you've made it past the plant. A town boat ramp is in the southwest corner of the harbor, with a long string of boat docks to the east. You must not only paddle parallel to these docks to return to Centennial Park, you must paddle past the ferry dock—which may or may not have a ferry sitting at it. If it does, paddle *far* behind its stern while keeping a close eye for its eventual departure.

Once you've left the power plant behind, navigated the boat docks, and passed the ferry at a safe distance, just another few hundred feet of paddling will have you back at the beach at Centennial Park, where you can load up your gear, change your clothes, and hit the town for some ice cream and fun.

◇ **SHUTTLE DIRECTIONS** To get to the put-in in Centennial Park, take I-495 (the Long Island Expressway) to Exit 64N (NY 112). Continue on NY 112 for 8.5 miles until it turns into NY 25A. Take NY 25A for an additional 1.5 miles to its end at Port Jefferson's ferry dock. Turn right at this point onto East Broadway, and continue 0.2 mile before turning left into the Port Jefferson Village Center parking lot. Travel partway around the traffic circle, taking the first right turn and following it past the Village Center. Continue down the dirt road, following the signs for Centennial Park. Look for the put-in at the far end of the dirt parking lot.

27 ROBINS ISLAND

◇ **OVERVIEW** On an island as densely populated and heavily developed as Long Island, finding large tracts of open land that have remained untouched by man is often hard to do. Amazingly, 435 such acres of land sit right in the middle of Peconic Bay. Because it is incredibly beautiful and it lies just a short distance offshore, this area, known as Robins Island, has become a very popular paddling destination.

It seems unlikely that an island that has had as many owners as this one could remain undeveloped for so long. Luckily, this is exactly what happened. Robins Island was first deeded to the Earl of Stirling, William Alexander, in 1635. The Earl then gave it to his attorney, James Farret, who in turn sold it to another man, Stephen Goodyear. Goodyear held on to the island for a couple of decades, but he too eventually sold it off to an interested buyer. Robins Island was then taken over by British forces during the American Revolution, after which it changed hands several more times. Incredibly, none of these owners altered the island to any great extent, allowing it to remain remarkably pristine and undisturbed.

Real estate developers did enter the picture in the late 1980s, seeking to build luxury homes on the island. The local government stepped in and attempted to protect Robins Island by purchasing it but was ultimately thwarted by intricacies of a legal nature. Thankfully, the island was eventually sold to Wall Street broker Louis Bacon, who is dedicated to preserving it and maintaining its ecological integrity. A few buildings have been constructed since Bacon bought the land, but he has also sought to remove invasive species, replace trees harvested for wood, and control the burgeoning populations of deer and other nuisance species.

Less than 1 mile from both the North and South forks, Robins Island is easily accessible by kayakers looking to enjoy its natural splendor for themselves. The island acts like an ill-fitting plug between the two forks, partially blocking the flow of water through Peconic Bay. As a result, it can have some serious tidal currents running along its northern and southern tips. For this reason, it's best to make crossings during slack tide. But once you're across, you'll feel as if you've paddled back into history, seeing the land as it was hundreds of years ago.

The 4-mile shoreline is dotted with glacial erratics of varying sizes, leading up to steep, sandy bluffs that can reach 30 feet high at some spots. Because of these steep slopes, little of the island's interior is visible, although its dense stands of oak and cedar trees are ever-visible and quite impressive. Red-tailed hawks can often be found gliding through the skies above, while geese, gulls, and terns are almost always abundant along the beaches. A healthy population of bank swallows nests in holes visible near the cliff tops.

When you consider all that Robins Island has to offer, it's no wonder that

Robins Island: Around the Island

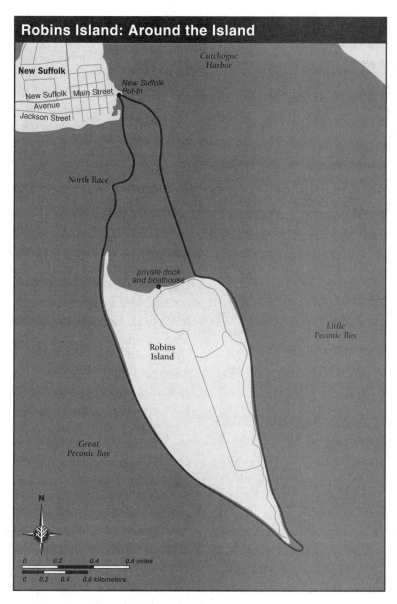

Cutchogue Harbor

New Suffolk

New Suffolk   Main Street
Avenue
Jackson Street

New Suffolk
Put-In

North Race

*private dock
and boathouse*

*Little
Peconic Bay*

Robins
Island

*Great
Peconic Bay*

N

0   0.2   0.4   0.6 miles

0   0.2   0.4   0.6 kilometers

it is often referred to as "The Jewel of the Peconic." Remember, though, that this jewel is privately owned and no trespassers are tolerated on its shores. Warning signs are posted around the island, and a patrol boat often circles its perimeter. By all means paddle to Robins Island, but make sure your kayak seat is comfortable—you won't be leaving it for the duration of your 6-mile trip.

USGS Quadrangles
SOUTHAMPTON (NY)

27 DESCRIPTION You should have a fairly good view of Robins Island and the crossing you're about to embark upon from your put-in in New Suffolk.

Around the Island

Level	3B
Distance	6 miles around
Time	3 hours
Navigable months	Year-round
Hazards	Open water
Portages	None
Rescue access	Difficult
Tidal conditions	Crossings best at slack tides
Scenery	C

Use this opportunity to look across, check out the water conditions before setting out, and decide in which direction you'll be rounding the island. I prefer to paddle counterclockwise during a flood (westward-flowing) tide and clockwise during an ebb (eastward-flowing) tide, though doing the opposite can work as well. It really comes down to personal preference, although slack tide—when little to no current is running—is obviously best.

To paddle the western side of Robins Island first, head south across the North Race, as the channel of water between you and the island is called, and point your boat toward the tip of the sandy spit that extends almost 0.5 mile from the island's northern shore. As you do, fix your eyes on the island for a decent view of its only dock, a boathouse, and a larger house farther inland. Get a good look at these structures, as they will be the only signs of civilization visible on your trip. Also keep an eye out for the island's small fleet of World War II–era beach-landing vessels, used to ferry people and supplies across the North Race. These unique vessels are great fun to watch.

Once you've finished paddling along the northern spit and are alongside Robins Island's mainland, you should see a small marsh to your left. Although it looks enticing, it's off-limits like the rest of the island. Fortunately, the water just offshore of the beach is not privately owned and is wonderful to paddle on.

The whole of Robins Island's western shore is undeveloped (as is its eastern shore), with only a 1.7-mile-long pebbly beach, a few large glacial erratics, and a pretty substantial bluff to show for itself. Keep looking at the bluff as you paddle in its shadow, and you should see a few small, sporadic holes near the top. These holes were created as nesting sites by bank swallows, which, if you're lucky, can be seen flitting about in search of their insect prey. If you could see inside of one of the holes, you'd find a tunnel anywhere from a few inches to a few feet long, with a small nest of straw and feathers lying at its end.

Keep gazing upwards toward the trees growing above the bluffs, and you may notice an interesting phenomenon. Because of the area's prevailing west winds, the growth of the trees atop the island have been

GPS COORDINATES

Put-in/take-out
N40° 59.493' W72° 28.230'
Tide station
New Suffolk, NY
N40° 59.502' W72° 28.302'

stunted. Their tops seem to be slanted toward the east, as if they're trying to escape the persistent breeze. Keep their shape in your head and compare it with that of the trees growing on the island's east side—you should see a difference. If your sight line drifts from the island's wonderfully pristine shore, you may glimpse the iconic windmill of the National Golf Links, across the bay in Southampton. That it can be seen at all demonstrates just how close Robins Island's southern tip is to Long Island's South Fork: less than 1 mile away.

After 3 miles of paddling, you'll reach the southern tip, which you'll have to round to gain access to the island's east side. Depending on the state of the tide, you may also have to face its current head-on as you turn east, although its effect will quickly diminish as you begin moving north. In just a few short strokes, you'll also

be sitting in the shadow of the island's bluffs once again, until you reach its northern tip.

As I mentioned earlier, the landscape of the island's east side differs from that of the west in a way that you may or may not notice, depending on how observant you've been. Here, on the downwind side of the island, the oak and cedar treetops seem a bit less stunted than on the opposite side, angled so as to put the least amount of resistance in front of the breeze.

Continue paddling and you'll reach Robins Island's north shore before you know it (the eastern shore is only 1.4 miles long). Once there, you should have a good sight line between your position and your take-out in New Suffolk, and you can begin the 1-mile crossing back to your car. You can also put this crossing off a bit if you want to paddle a bit closer to the island's boat dock and check out the large

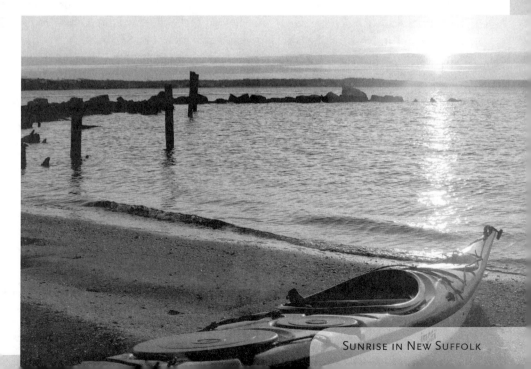

SUNRISE IN NEW SUFFOLK

house that sits nearby. Just remember to respect the residents' privacy by not paddling too close.

◇ **SHUTTLE DIRECTIONS** To get to the put-in in New Suffolk, take NY 25 into the village of Mattituck and turn right onto New Suffolk Avenue (left if coming from the east). Travel 3.5 miles on New Suffolk Avenue and look for the beach at its end. Drop your boat and gear off at the water's edge, and park anywhere there's room along the shoulder of First Street.

---

28 SAG HARBOR

◇ **OVERVIEW** How many places can you think of that saw action during both the Revolutionary War and War of 1812, were mentioned in *Moby-Dick,* are currently home to a number of celebrities, and are named after a tuber-producing plant? I can think of only one: Sag Harbor.

The town was first settled by Europeans sometime in the early 18th century, and yes, it was named after a plant, specifically *Apios americana,* or the groundnut. How did the settlers get *Sag* from *groundnut*? They used a shortened version of the native Algonquin name for the plant, *Sagabon.* Once the naming was taken care of, these men and women set about establishing a port in their new town. Fortunately, their port quickly grew in size, and by the end of the 18th century it had become an international port of entry for the colony of New York. Some say, in fact, that it rivaled New York City's harbor in ships' tonnage.

Such a prosperous seaport also enabled the whaling industry to come quite easily to the harbor, reaching its peak in the mid-1800s before its eventual collapse a few decades later. The industry's effects on the town were long-lasting, however, and many of its artifacts remain today. Paying homage to those who worked, and perhaps lost their lives, in the whaling business are the Sag Harbor Whaling Museum, the Old Whalers' Church, and the Broken Mast Monument.

To this day, Sag Harbor has managed to retain most of its seaport-town appeal, although its square-rigged sailing ships have all been replaced by megayachts and powerboats. The sounds of the waves and smells of the sea are still present, however, and have helped make the town the popular tourist destination it is. Sailors, fishermen, families, and the well-heeled come to Sag Harbor to enjoy its charm. It's definitely my favorite South Fork town.

As one can imagine, a harbor that caters to large boats and their owners usually has few amenities set aside for kayakers. Sag Harbor is no exception: the boat ramps are usually off-limits and waterfront parking can be nonexistent, especially on sunny summer days. Paddlers do have one spot to launch from, though. The village beach, adjacent to the "Long Wharf," is an excellent put-in that's free and open to everyone. Look for it behind the large wooden windmill, and park as close

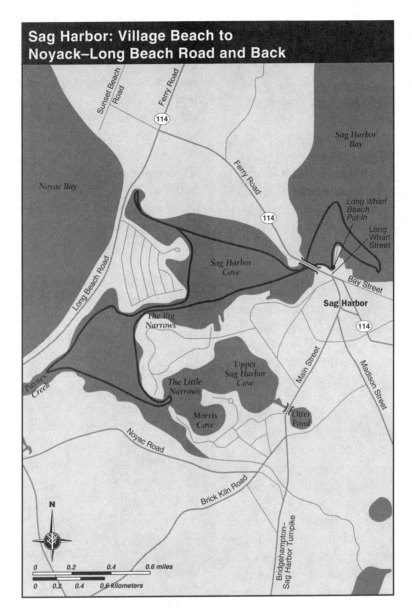

Sag Harbor: Village Beach to Noyack–Long Beach Road and Back

to it as you can. Getting to the water may require a bit of a walk and several trips to transfer all your gear, but rest assured—the effort is well worth it.

USGS Quadrangles GREENPORT (NY), SAG HARBOR (NY)

28 **DESCRIPTION** Paddlers have a multitude of options to choose from once they've launched from the village beach. Cedar Point and its lighthouse are only a 3-mile paddle to the northeast. Heading 3 miles to the northwest brings you to Shelter Island's southern shore. And the beautiful waters of Northwest Harbor lie less than 2 miles to the east. My favorite destination is the series of coves to the southwest,

Village Beach to Noyack–Long Beach Road and Back

Level	2B
Distance	6.2 miles round-trip
Time	2–3 hours
Navigable months	Year-round
Hazards	Boat traffic
Portages	None
Rescue access	Easy
Tidal conditions	Any
Scenery	B

although I always make it a point to paddle through the harbor a bit first and get a good look at the amazing boats that are almost always there.

If you'd like to do the same, head north after hitting the water, paddle around the pier known as Long Wharf, and the whole of Sag Harbor will open before you. During spring and summer, hundreds of boats can be seen floating on their moorings inside the long stone breakwater. But it's along the harbor front where you'll find the truly amazing boats. Summer brings the rich and famous, and their megayachts, to Sag Harbor. These huge vessels dwarf kayaks, and most other boats for that matter, but they possess a measure of beauty and grace despite their immense size. If you check out these maritime wonders, do so carefully—you wouldn't want to find yourself directly underneath one of these behemoths as its engines are firing.

More docks sit a few hundred feet to the east of the megayacht docks. The boats moored here are smaller but sometimes just as impressive as their bigger cousins. Among other celebrities, Billy Joel and Jimmy Buffett own boats that can sometimes be seen here. Famous people aside, the harbor is almost always a fascinating place to paddle and boat-watch. But when the crowds have gotten to be too much, head toward the Route 114 Bridge and Sag Harbor's back coves, just 0.5 mile to the west.

Pass under the large bridge and by a small marina, and you'll be paddling in the first of three main coves. Aptly named Sag Harbor Cove, it's roughly oval, although it narrows a bit at its western end. You'll notice that the cove's shores are lined with houses and private docks. Much the same is true for the two subsequent coves as well. This development may deter some paddlers looking to commune with nature. They would surely miss out, though, as the waters shelter a wide assortment of birds and other creatures.

Ospreys have been known to soar in the skies above, while great blue herons and great egrets commonly stalk the shallow waters in search of prey. Common terns can often be seen flitting about, diving into the water on occasion to grab a quick meal. Diamondback terrapins also spend a good deal of time in the waters of the coves, poking their heads out from time to

GPS Coordinates

Put-in/take-out
N41° 00.184' W72° 17.768'
Tide station
Sag Harbor, NY
N41° 00.198' W72° 17.802'

time to catch a breath. Paddle here between late fall and winter, and you'll see a completely different assortment of birds: buffleheads, red-breasted mergansers, and common mergansers, to name just a few.

Follow Sag Harbor Cove to its westernmost tip, where a small yet secluded salt marsh sits undisturbed. From here you can portage over the rocky border of the marsh and across Long Beach Road, gaining access to Noyack Bay. In fact, the lure of Long Beach's sands, and its ice-cream trucks, has drawn many a paddler away from the cove. For those that have resisted the temptation, however, the next cove can be found southwest of Sag Harbor Cove, through a narrow stretch of water appropriately named "The Big Narrows."

Although this cove seems not to have been named, it contains two arms, to the southwest and southeast, that have been. The former, Paynes Creek, is only about 0.3 mile long. The latter, known as The Little Narrows, ultimately leads into the last of the large coves, Upper Sag Harbor Cove. Like the other coves, this one is dotted with houses along its length, but it also sports a somewhat unique feature. A small creek along the cove's southeastern corner leads to a small body of water known as Otter Pond. Despite sitting in the middle of a suburban development, the pond has retained a good deal of undisturbed shoreline and is often a good place to observe wading birds and ducks. After exiting Otter Pond and exploring the rest of Upper Sag Harbor Cove's shoreline, turn around and head back to your put-in, 1.5 miles away.

◇ **SHUTTLE DIRECTIONS** To get to the put-in at Sag Harbor, take NY 27 into the town of Bridgehampton. Turn left onto Bridgehampton–Sag Harbor Turnpike if coming from the west, right if coming from the east. Continue north for 3.4 miles, at which time Bridgehampton–Sag Harbor Turnpike becomes Main Street. Take Main Street 1.2 miles farther north into Sag Harbor. Look for the village beach in front of the windmill. You may launch your boat there and park along Long Wharf, if you're lucky enough to find a spot. Otherwise, park along the roads of the village or in the municipal lot.

---

29 SEBONAC CREEK

◇ **OVERVIEW** In the town of Southampton is a body of water so amazing, it may very well be the prettiest spot to paddle on all of Long Island. Called Sebonac Creek, it actually consists of three separate creeks and two small bays, all of which connect to form a paddler's paradise. Natural beauty, little development, protected waters, abundant wildlife, and miles of shoreline—few other places I have paddled even come close.

As is often the case on Long Island, Sebonac Creek and its environs were once the domain of Native Americans. In this instance, it was the Shinnecock tribe who knew the area's value as a

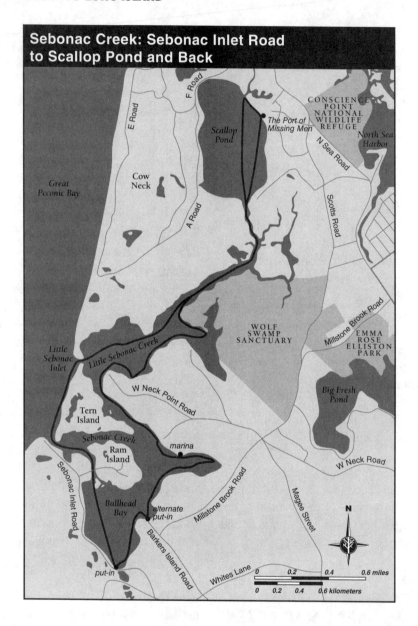

Sebonac Creek: Sebonac Inlet Road to Scallop Pond and Back

source of food, harvesting scallops, clams, oysters, and many species of fish from the creek's productive waters. The European colonists also recognized the value of the land as they began heavily hunting its deer and waterfowl, fishing its waters, and cutting down its trees for firewood and

building materials. In fact, most of the trees in the area had been cut down by the end of the 18th century, creating a landscape very different from what the original inhabitants knew.

Thankfully, visitors to Sebonac Creek today may find it hard to imagine that clear-cutting and overhunting occurred at all. This is due in part to the area's fertility and also the conservation efforts of its more-recent residents. Besides a few private homes and a nationally renowned golf course along its southern borders, most of the Sebonac Creek estuary is contained within a park, sanctuary, refuge, or preserve. Indeed, an examination of the area using Google Earth reveals just how much undeveloped land exists in the area.

And where there is open land, there is often a great deal of natural diversity. Sebonac's vast salt marsh supports a wide array of waterfowl and wading birds, from black ducks and green herons to snowy egrets. Terns nest in large numbers here, as do ospreys and piping plovers. With the coming of winter, many migratory waterfowl like mergansers and buffleheads also become commonplace. Not as obvious as birds, but just as important ecologically, are three plant rare species that grow in the estuary. The Nature Conservancy has identified salt-marsh aster, marsh pink, and slender blue flag (a type of iris) within its boundaries.

It is extremely fortunate that the area around Sebonac Creek has been preserved and protected. Even better, its unspoiled beauty is easily accessible to bird-watchers, nature-lovers, and

paddlers alike. In fact, paddlers will find a multitude of potential put-ins along Sebonac Creek. Many of these are open to everyone, even non–Southampton residents. The most convenient put-in, however, is on the southernmost part of the creek, off Sebonac Inlet Road.

USGS Quadrangles
SOUTHAMPTON (NY)

29 **DESCRIPTION** With such an amazing view from the put-in, it's hard to decide which direction to set out in when paddling Sebonac Creek. With little more than salt-marsh-lined shores, calm and protected water, and a charming windmill standing in the distance (albeit it on a golf course and not a farm), both shores look equally enticing, and they are. Paddling along the eastern shore provides the more direct route north to Scallop Pond, though, which may influence your choice.

Once you've made your decision and launched your boat, you'll be paddling on the small body of water

Sebonac Inlet Road to Scallop Pond and Back

Level	1B
Distance	8 miles round-trip
Time	3–4 hours
Navigable months	Year-round
Hazards	None
Portages	None
Rescue access	Limited
Tidal conditions	3 hours before or after high tide
Scenery	A+

GPS COORDINATES

Put-in/take-out
N40° 54.459' W72° 26.663'
Tide station
Shinnecock Canal, NY
N40° 54.000' W72° 30.000'

known as Bullhead Bay. Even from the seat of your kayak, it should be truly obvious just how little development there is along the shores. Sure, a dead-end road appears at the water's edge just 0.4 mile north of the put-in (itself a very convenient put-in), and a beautiful house sits a bit farther north, just across the cove from the road. Otherwise, all that remains is the lush, green vegetation that composes the marsh here.

As in most salt marshes, *Spartina alterniflora* (smooth cordgrass) is the predominant plant here, growing at the water's edge. Its shorter cousin, *Spartina patens* (salt-meadow cordgrass), grows a bit higher up on land. The invasive plant known as phragmites grows just beyond the spartina grasses, with marsh elder occupying the highest and driest parts of the marsh. Here on Sebonac Creek, large oak and maple trees provide the

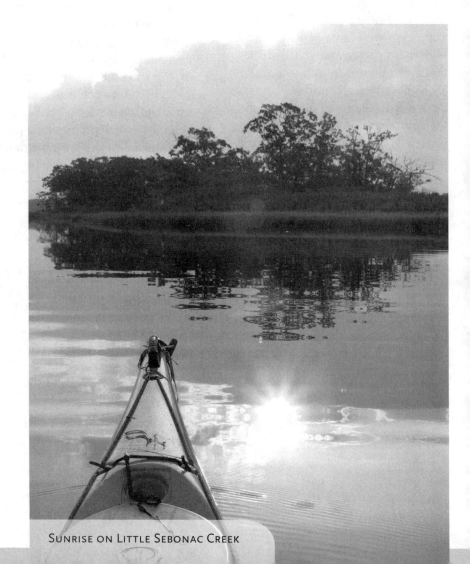

SUNRISE ON LITTLE SEBONAC CREEK

final boundary of the area, lining the edges of the marsh and separating it from the mainland.

After 0.5 mile of paddling along-side these marsh plants, you'll come to Ram Island and a small mooring field of boats to its immediate right. Most mooring fields are associated with a marina, and this one is no exception. In this case, the mooring field and marina sit on the northern shore of the small cove to the east, with a scattering of houses nearby to keep them company.

Paddle a bit farther north along Sebonac Creek, and a low-lying, tri-angular piece of land known as Tern Island will come in to view on the left. The island is a fabulous place to paddle, with a tidal creek on its eastern shore that leads to a small pond in its center. It may be best left for the return trip, however, especially if Scallop Pond is your ultimate goal. If this is the case, skirt around the island to the right and continue your paddle north.

The narrow path of Sebonac Creek turns sharply east immediately after you pass Tern Island and enters a much wider stretch of water, ironi-cally called Little Sebonac Creek. With all powerboats left behind and all but a few isolated homes dotting the very distant shore, this portion of the estuary is where the fun really begins. Have your binoculars out and camera ready. The last time I paddled here, I spied many diamondback terrapins poking their heads out of the water, as well as more than a few ospreys fly-ing overhead or sitting in their nests. Least terns (the ones with the yellow bills) are also common here, as are

great and snowy egrets and great blue herons. Lucky paddlers may even get to see a white-tailed deer feeding along the shoreline or a muskrat swimming across a tidal creek.

You'll eventually reach a fork when paddling northeast up Little Sebonac Creek. To the right lies a fairly large cove with some houses on its south-ern shore and nothing but salt marsh everywhere else. Exploring every inch of its 1 mile of shoreline is well worth the effort, especially for those who can't get enough of the natural beauty of the area. The left fork leads to West Neck Creek, which stretches a slender path through almost 1 mile of additional salt marsh before emptying into Scallop Pond. Before it reaches the pond, though, it winds past a small handful of duck blinds, complete with active osprey nests on their roofs, and a fairly large creek on the right that runs 0.5 mile to the northeast before coming to an end.

Once Scallop Pond is finally reached, a most unique destination lies waiting. Just 0.5 mile to the north stands the only building on the pond: an estate known as The Port of Miss-ing Men. Built in 1926 as a hunting lodge for socialite Millicent Rogers, it supposedly gained its name when a rudder from a shipwrecked vessel was found on the property. With this maritime theme in mind, the Rog-ers family even had the basement of the house constructed and painted to look like the stern of a sailing ship. The entire estate once consisted of upwards of 1,200 acres but now encompasses much less. Its gran-deur has not faded a bit, though.

Just across the pond from The Port of Missing Men sits another large tract of land, this one 540 acres large. Also once part of the Rogers family's original plot, this piece of property has now been designated as a greenway for wildlife, protected from development indefinitely. Examining the land, known as the Cow Neck Peninsula, on Google Earth shows just how large and unspoiled the area really is. From a conservation standpoint, its protected status is a true blessing.

As you head back down West Neck Creek, and eventually into Little Sebonac Creek, Little Sebonac Inlet soon becomes visible. This tiny gap between Cow Neck and Tern Island may sometimes be closed due to weather and tide conditions. But when it's open, it provides easy access to Peconic Bay, with Robins Island little more than 2 miles to the north. Exiting through its gap also enables you to round Tern Island on the bay side, where you'll find yet another scenic paddling spot.

As its name suggests, Tern Island is *the* place to see the tiny white birds in the Sebonac estuary. Likewise, the diminutive piping plover is also very common along the island's shores. The Long Island nesting habitats of these two endangered birds are most often protected during spring and summer, and the beaches of Tern Island are no exception. Give them a wide berth when paddling, and only observe the nesting birds from afar.

The outer side of Tern Island runs 0.5 mile south before ending at Sebonac Inlet. On the opposite side of this wider opening sits another potential put-in, at the end of Sebonac Inlet Road. Returning to Sebonac Creek through the inlet soon brings you to Ram Island's western shore, where a small wooden bridge spans the creek and separates the island from the mainland. Once you pass beneath the bridge, the half-mile crossing of Bullhead Bay is all that stands between you and your car.

✧ **SHUTTLE DIRECTIONS** To get to the put-in on Sebonac Inlet Road, take NY 27 into the town of Southampton and turn left onto Tuckahoe Road (right if coming from the east). Continue north on Tuckahoe Road 1 mile, until it ends at an intersection with Sebonac Road. Turn left onto Sebonac Road and take it 0.25 mile to a fork with Sebonac Inlet Road. Bear right at the fork, following Sebonac Inlet Road 0.6 mile until you reach the water. Park anywhere along the guardrail on the small bridge crossing the creek, and launch from either shore.

30 SETAUKET HARBOR

✧ **OVERVIEW** Setauket Harbor is a quaint body of water with a storied history and a healthy dose of small-town charm. In the town of Setauket, nestled between Stony Brook and Port Jefferson, the harbor's protected waters draw fishermen, clammers, sailors, bird-watchers, and of course paddlers. In fact, this is my personal favorite

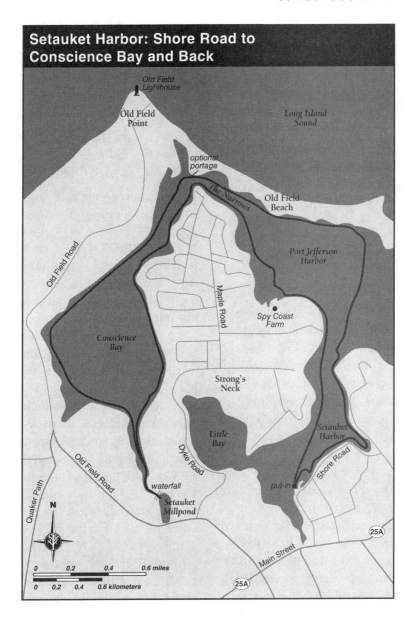

Setauket Harbor: Shore Road to Conscience Bay and Back

Old Field Lighthouse

Old Field Point

Long Island Sound

optional portage

The Narrows

Old Field Beach

Port Jefferson Harbor

Old Field Road

Maple Road

Spy Coast Farm

Conscience Bay

Strong's Neck

Setauket Harbor

Little Bay

Old Field Road

Dyke Road

Shore Road

Quaker Path

waterfall

put-in

Setauket Millpond

N

25A

Main Street

25A

| 0 | 0.2 | 0.4 | 0.6 miles |

| 0 | 0.2 | 0.4 | 0.6 kilometers |

place to kayak. Nine paddles out of ten, I am on Setauket Harbor.

The harbor and its adjacent town were named after the area's original inhabitants, the Setalcott Indians. Europeans soon entered the picture and, in 1655, purchased the land for an amazingly small assortment of axes, needles, knives, lead, and clothing, thus creating the very first European settlement in the town of Brookhaven. The area's development continued throughout the late 17th and early 18th centuries. With good soil, a protected harbor, and abundant shellfish and finfish, Setauket housed a good number of farmers, fishermen, and seamen. During the Revolutionary War, it became home to an important part of George Washington's now-famous spy ring.

With the end of the war and the dawn of a new century, Setauket Harbor became a logical place to begin building ships. The industry quickly flourished, ultimately producing many ships, the largest of which was the *Adorna,* at 1,460 tons. As the shipbuilders closed shop, other industries came to Setauket, including a piano factory and a large rubber factory. These also shut down eventually, leaving room for the mom-and-pop shops that have helped Setauket retain its small-town feel.

Thankfully, Setauket's past has not been relegated to the history books. It is visible almost everywhere one looks. A number of the town's residents live in historic homes. Local museums showcase 18th- and 19th-century living. There is an annual Setalcott Indian pow-wow. And one of the local elementary schools celebrates Setauket Founders' Day each spring.

Paddling on Setauket Harbor reveals even more history. Cruising its shores lets you see the remains of the shipbuilding industry that prospered here. The shorefront property that was once used by the spy ring still exists today as a horse farm. Even the remnants of an old wooden bridge, once used by schooners to unload their cargo of coal for the factories, can be found where it once crossed Setauket Harbor.

As for launching a kayak, there's no better spot than the public beach on Shore Road. Parking is free and easy, although conditions are largely tide-dependent. The beach becomes little more than a vast mudflat at low tide, making paddling almost impossible. In such cases, the dock at the end of the pier provides an alternative, although it may be a bit high off the water for some. In any case, Setauket Harbor is—and will surely remain—a great place to paddle. I'll see you there!

USGS Quadrangles
PORT JEFFERSON (NY)

30 **DESCRIPTION** You have several paddling options when launching from the beach on Shore Road. Turning 180 degrees south and heading down the small creek for 0.3 mile will bring you to the dock of the local kayak outfitter and to the parking lot of a locally famous delicatessen. Indeed, many people begin their trip this way, picking up lunch before heading out into the harbor. Alternately, you can head almost due west from the beach and enter a small piece of water aptly called Little Bay. Quite shallow and muddy at low tide, Little Bay is a popular water-skiing spot when water levels are higher. It's also the location of the remains of a bridge crossing to Strong's Neck: look to the south just as you enter Little Bay, and the stone foundation of one end of the bridge is visible on the shore. The usual paddling option, though, is to turn east

GPS COORDINATES

Put-in/take-out
N40° 56.891' W73° 06.160'
Tide station
Port Jefferson Harbor Entrance, NY
N40° 58.257' W73° 05.588'

Shore Road to Conscience Bay and Back

Level	2B
Distance	9 miles round-trip
Time	4 hours
Navigable months	Year-round
Hazards	Boat traffic
Portages	1 (optional)
Rescue access	Easy
Tidal conditions	4 hours before or after high tide
Scenery	A

from the beach and begin heading out into the harbor itself.

Many of the houses lining the harbor's edge there are historic, built by ship's captains or builders. In fact, a few of the larger buildings were once part of the shipyards themselves. A few relics and skeletons of old wooden sailing ships can even be seen at low tide in Scott's Cove, the small cove just over 0.5 mile from the beach. Google Earth has some pretty good images of this area, which is worth a look.

More homes line the waterfront north of Scott's Cove, although these are more modern in design. Their residents also have their own beach a few hundred feet north of the cove; it's private property, however, so landing is prohibited. A smaller beach, on a spit of land just a bit farther north, is open to any paddler. Its location makes it ideal for a rest or snack stop. Look west across the harbor at this point— one of the homes of the prominent Strong family is visible through the trees (look for the yellow house with

four chimneys through the trees). The house, named The Cedars, was built in 1879 atop the peninsula that has since been named Strong's Neck, after the family that called it home.

The waters of Setauket Harbor end and those of Port Jefferson Harbor begin 1.25 miles northeast of the beach on Shore Road. Here, paddlers again have some options to choose from. Turning around and heading back into Setauket Harbor is one possibility, as is continuing along the eastern shore into Port Jefferson Harbor. Another option is to head northwest to The Narrows, a section of water that leads into Conscience Bay. My favorite choice, though, is to head due north from Setauket Harbor and cross the 0.6 mile to Old Field Beach. It's usually not too crowded and is excellent for picnicking, swimming, or bird-watching. Great blue herons, great egrets, common terns, sanderlings, and the occasional oystercatcher or two are usually seen strutting or flitting along the pebbly shoreline on Old Field Beach.

Anyone who goes for a walk here is also likely to see a plant that's unusual for this area. Long Island's only indigenous cactus, the prickly pear, grows in relatively large amounts on higher ground here. Quite small and low to the ground, it produces a somewhat sweet, fleshy fruit that is exceedingly edible. In fact, many people make it a point to pick prickly pears each fall to use in jams and other recipes. Visit Old Field Beach in October to help yourself to these reddish-purple pears. Watch your hands and feet when picking, though—they don't call it prickly pear for nothing.

You can paddle along Old Field Beach for almost 1 mile, hugging the shore and staying out of the way of boats both moored and moving. Eventually, the thin strip of land meets mainland Old Field just after The Narrows. From this point, Conscience Bay sits just a stone's throw away, beckoning paddlers to explore its waters. More-adventurous souls may choose another option, however, and carry their boats over Old Field Beach before it meets the mainland, then relaunch on Long Island Sound. The Old Field Lighthouse to the west and the Port Jefferson Harbor entrance to the east are just two potential destinations that this portage opens.

Those choosing to paddle Conscience Bay instead of setting out on the sound need only paddle 0.5 mile through its narrow entrance before the round bay spreads before them. At less than 1 mile across, Conscience Bay is quite small. In fact, you can see just about every nook and cranny of its shoreline from every other point on it. Dotted with houses both large and small and quite shallow, the bay proper contains little in the way of attention-grabbing features. Heading due south from its entrance, however, brings paddlers to an amazing spot worth a visit. A tiny, narrow cove points southward from that corner of the bay and ends at an old gristmill and waterfall in a beautiful place called Frank Melville Memorial Park. You must negotiate a tight, shallow path through phragmites before reaching the waterfall, though, and you can do so only when water levels are high enough. But with a bit of luck and a lot of persistence, you can paddle right to the base of the falls.

After paddling throughout Conscience Bay and its 1.5 miles of shoreline, then passing through The Narrows once more, paddlers will be back on Setauket Harbor. Staying to the south here instead of off Old Field Beach affords views of a stunning piece of property on an historic parcel of land. This large horse farm, Spy Coast Farm, sits on land that was once the hunting and fishing land of the Setalcott Indians. It's also said to be where a famous Revolutionary War patriot, Anna Smith Strong, played an important part in George Washington's spy ring. Strong would hang a certain number of petticoats in a particular order on her clothesline near the water's edge—thus passing on messages to other spies about the British troops in the area.

Once you've passed the lush green grass and galloping horses of Spy Coast Farm, the beach will curve to the south and lead directly to the main portion of the harbor, where the put-in on Shore Road sits just 1 mile farther.

✥ **SHUTTLE DIRECTIONS** To get to the put-in on Shore Road, take I-495 (the Long Island Expressway) to Exit 62N (CR 97). Take CR 97 (Nicolls Road) north 9.7 miles, until it ends in Stony Brook. Turn right onto NY 25A and continue east 1.6 miles. Just past the Se-Port Deli, turn left onto Shore Road and continue north 0.3 mile. Look for the beach and parking pier as the road curves to the right.

31 SHELTER ISLAND AND MASHOMACK PRESERVE

◇ **OVERVIEW** The Mashomack Preserve on Shelter Island's south shore is one of the most pristine and beautiful areas on all of Long Island. Originally part of the Manhanset Indians' hunting and fishing territory, it got its name from the Native American word meaning "Where they go by water." The natives enjoyed exclusive rights to this very productive land for quite some time, until their chief, Pogatticut, sold all of Shelter Island to a sugar merchant named Nathaniel Sylvester in 1653. Nathaniel's son, Giles, inherited the property when his father died in

1680 and began selling off parts of it 13 years later. The land that now includes the preserve was among the parcels sold, purchased by the Nicoll family. Amazingly, they retained ownership of Mashomack for the next 250 years.

The land exchanged hands a few times after the Nicolls parted with it, until it was finally picked up by the Mashomack Fish and Game Club in the mid-1900s. Because the land hadn't been developed by any of its previous owners (besides a few scattered buildings), it had remained almost as unspoiled and biologically productive as when the Manhansets lived there—a fact the new owners took full advantage of. Mashomack's beauty also attracted the attention of The Nature Conservancy, an organization that seeks to protect natural

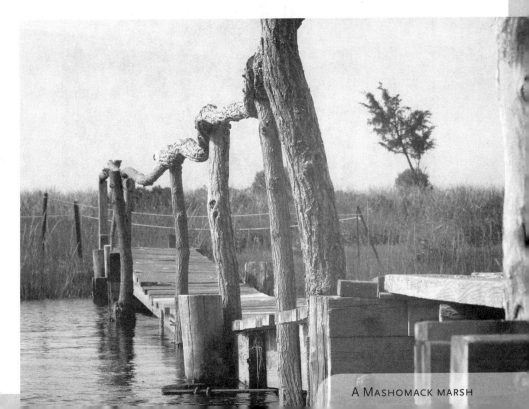

A MASHOMACK MARSH

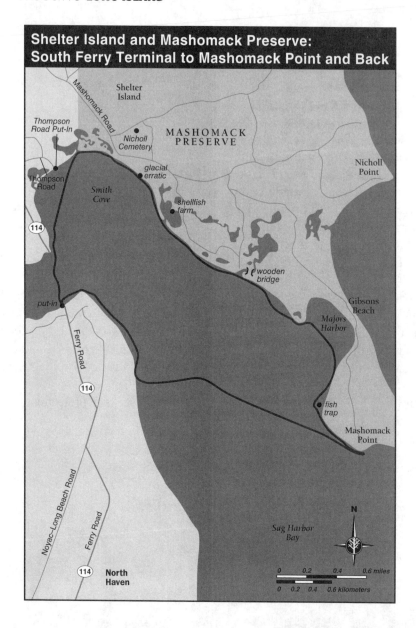

**Shelter Island and Mashomack Preserve:
South Ferry Terminal to Mashomack Point and Back**

Shelter Island

Mashomack Road

Thompson Road Put-In

Nicholl Cemetery

MASHOMACK PRESERVE

Nicholl Point

glacial erratic

Thompson Road

Smith Cove

shellfish farm

114

wooden bridge

Gibsons Beach

put-in

Majors Harbor

Ferry Road

114

fish trap

Mashomack Point

Noyac–Long Beach Road

Ferry Road

114 **North Haven**

Sag Harbor Bay

N

0   0.2   0.4   0.6 miles

0   0.2   0.4   0.6 kilometers

biodiversity by purchasing and protecting unique and endangered pieces of land. Luckily, the conservancy was able to purchase the Mashomack property from the hunting club for $10.6 million when its real-estate-development scheme collapsed, and thus was able to protect it forever.

The preserve today encompasses almost 2,100 acres, with an incredible 10 miles of shoreline. Within its boundaries exists one of the largest breeding populations of ospreys on the East Coast, nesting colonies of both piping plovers and least terns, and a pine-swamp habitat that has been declared "a freshwater wetland of unique local importance" by New York State. It boasts vast salt marshes, tidal creeks, dense forests, and an immense variety of wildlife.

Visiting the preserve and enjoying its incredible beauty is quite easy to do. Open most days of the week year-round, it offers guided hikes and bird-watching walks fairly regularly. Check out **bit.ly/d853rZ** on the Web for more information on these activities. While Mashomack does not allow launching of canoes or kayaks from preserve property, its shores cry out to be explored by boat—recall that its name translates to "Where they go by water." The preserve is easily reached by launching from the beach next to Shelter Island's South Ferry dock or from the Shelter Island town put-in on Thompson Road.

USGS Quadrangles GREENPORT (NY)

31 **DESCRIPTION** To paddle along the pristine shoreline of the Masho-mack Preserve, you must first cross the small stretch of water between North Haven and Shelter Island. Although it may seem straightforward and easy, the 0.3-mile crossing can be difficult at times, with wind, tidal currents, and the comings and go-ings of the South Ferry conspiring to make your trip a bit of a challenge. If you should arrive at the ferry terminal in North Haven and find conditions unsuitable for crossing, a better and safer option is to take the ferry across to Shelter Island and launch from the put-in on Thompson Road instead. Under such circumstances, purchas-ing the $15 round-trip ticket will be well worth the trouble it saves.

South Ferry Terminal to Mashomack Point and Back

Level	3B
Distance	8.8 miles round-trip
Time	4 hours
Navigable months	Year-round
Hazards	Boat traffic, open water
Portages	None
Rescue access	Limited
Tidal conditions	Any
Scenery	A+

Whether you've paddled across or taken the ferry to the island and launched from its south shore, you'll be floating in a crescent-shaped cove known as Smith Cove, named after industrialist Francis Marion Smith, one of the island's prominent 19th- and early-20th-century residents. The Mashomack Preserve's boundary lies near the center of the cove. At this point you'll probably notice the signs posted along the beach prohibiting boat landing. As unfortunate as this prohibition is, paddlers must re-member that the preserve is part of a unique and fragile environment that needs protecting. Keeping our boats off its beaches and out of its creeks seem such small things to do to help

GPS COORDINATES

Put-in/take-out
N41° 02.370' W72° 18.931'
Tide station
Sag Harbor, NY
N41° 00.198' W72° 17.802'

ensure its survival. Besides, there is much to see along the beach from the seat of a kayak. Simply turn your bow to the east, begin paddling, and get ready to marvel at the splendor that is Mashomack.

A small break on the shore is easy to spot near the center of Smith Cove. Gaze down the small creek that flows there, and you should catch a glimpse of a series of saltwater ponds ringed with oak and maple trees. Were you able to paddle deeper among these ponds, you'd see that spartina grass grows far and wide throughout. Ospreys rest on branches overhead. Shorebirds run up and down the tiny beach. And juvenile fish school in the protected waters. To say the spot is pristine would be an understatement. Jaw-droppingly, unbelievably beautiful is more like it.

If you can manage to tear yourself away from this amazing view, head back out to Smith Cove and continue paddling southeast along its shore. As you head farther south, keep an eye out for an interesting geologic feature just a dozen or so feet offshore: a large erratic, or boulder, that was deposited by a glacier millions of years ago. More fascinating, though, is the fact that it split into two, most likely as a result of water that continuously seeped into cracks in the boulder and froze. Get a good look at this natural wonder, then paddle 0.75 mile farther to another tidal creek. Like the previous creek in Smith Cove, this one also leads to a series of saltwater ponds that are equally beautiful, and equally off-limits. Unlike the first creek, this one leads to a small shellfish farm that

was established by The Nature Conservancy to help restore native populations of clams, oysters, and scallops.

Beyond this shellfish farm, you'll notice that the shoreline has begun to curve slightly to the east. With this curve comes a decision: Do you turn around and head back to your car, a little over 1 mile away? If you've had your fill of the wonders of Mashomack, then yes, this is the way to go. Or do you continue following the shoreline as it curves south, with Mashomack Point as your ultimate destination? If you still want more stunning scenery, then paddle on.

By this point of the trip, you should have a good view of the peninsula you're headed toward. Incidentally, you should also be able to see much of Sag Harbor's waterfront if you look due south. On a spring or summer day, you can probably see a few megayachts sitting at its docks as well. Follow Mashomack's shore for an additional 0.5 mile, and a small cove named Majors Harbor will appear on your left. Hug its beach or cut a straight line across its width. Either way, once on the other side you'll be paddling alongside the teardrop-shaped peninsula that ends at Mashomack Point.

See the wooden stakes and mesh netting stretching out from the beach about halfway down the peninsula's western side? This is a fish trap, designed to block a fish's path and force it to swim farther offshore. Unfortunately for the fish, that usually means getting caught in the wide catch area and becoming either bait or dinner. Leave the trap for the fish, giving it a wide berth as you paddle around its offshore end. Paddle just 0.5 mile farther, and the small piece of land called Mashomack Point will be at your side.

Should you find yourself sitting on the point with more time and energy at your disposal, round it and head to the Cedar Point lighthouse, just 1 mile away. You might also want to paddle through the tidal estuary that runs through the center of the peninsula. Both would make excellent side trips. I usually choose to end my trip here, though, and either retrace my paddle strokes back up the coast or head west and cross over to North Haven, a bit over 2 miles distant. Obviously, such a crossing is largely weather-dependent, and you should do it only when conditions are ideal.

◇ **SHUTTLE DIRECTIONS** To get to the put-in in North Haven, take NY 27 into the town of Bridgehampton. Turn left onto Bridgehampton–Sag Harbor Turnpike if coming from the west, right if coming from the east. Continue north 3.4 miles, at which time Bridgehampton–Sag Harbor Turnpike becomes Main Street. Take Main Street 1.2 miles farther north into the village of Sag Harbor, where it will turn into NY 114. Take NY 114 out of Sag Harbor and you will reach a traffic circle in 1.2 miles. Take the first right turn off the circle and continue north on NY 114. You will reach Shelter Island's south ferry dock in 2 miles. Park in any open space on the left side of the road, immediately before the dock.

32 SHINNECOCK BAY

◇ **OVERVIEW** Shinnecock Bay, on Long Island's East End, holds a special place in my heart. Long famed as a source of shellfish and finfish, it is also a vital wintering ground for harbor and gray seals, an amazingly productive estuary, a nesting area for dozens of species of shorebirds, a summer home of juvenile sea turtles, and an important nursery for a wide variety of marine invertebrates such as clams, oysters, and crabs. Whales and dolphins have been known to swim and feed just offshore. Ospreys nest among its vast salt marshes. Even a tropical fish or two can be found here after being carried up the coast by the Gulf Stream. Naturally speaking, Shinnecock Bay is truly remarkable.

Little about the bay has changed since it was first inhabited by the Shinnecock people thousands of years ago. These natives fished its waters for bluefish, bass, and other important food species. They harvested clams, oysters, and mussels from its bottom and became well known as producers of high-quality wampum made from the shells of its bivalves. They even hunted whales that swam beyond its shores. When Europeans came to the Shinnecock area centuries later, they too found the area bountiful and productive. Benjamin Franklin Thompson wrote in his 1839 book *History of Long Island,* "This beautiful expanse of water has long been celebrated for the excellence and variety of its marine productions. The clams found here are

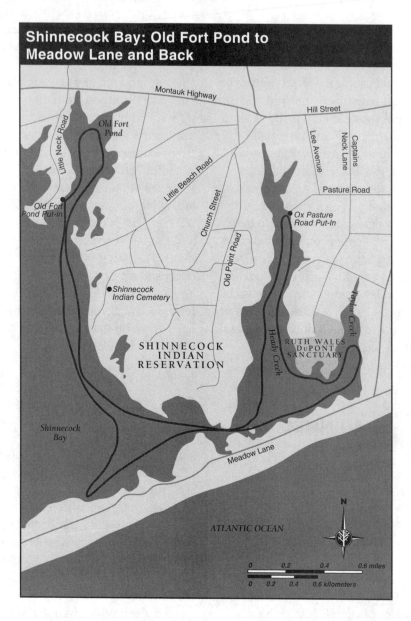

Shinnecock Bay: Old Fort Pond to Meadow Lane and Back

Montauk Highway

Hill Street

Little Neck Road

Old Fort Pond

Lee Avenue

Captains Neck Lane

Pasture Road

Old Fort Pond Put-In

Little Beach Road

Church Street

Ox Pasture Road Put-In

Old Point Road

Shinnecock Indian Cemetery

Taylor Creek

SHINNECOCK INDIAN RESERVATION

Heady Creek

RUTH WALES DuPONT SANCTUARY

Shinnecock Bay

Meadow Lane

ATLANTIC OCEAN

N

0   0.2   0.4   0.6 miles

0   0.2   0.4   0.6 kilometers

of a superior quality, and so abundant as to afford almost constant employment for about fifty persons." The English also reaped the benefits of the bay's extensive supplies of fish, hunted its waterfowl, and used its marshes as grazing land. In short, they appreciated its resources as much as the Native Americans did.

Things on Shinnecock Bay remained the same for many more decades, until one fateful day in 1938 when a massive hurricane—the worst weather disaster to hit the Northeast in modern times—smashed into Long Island and broke a hole through the barrier beach that separated the bay from the Atlantic. In an unexpected upside to the hurricane's destruction, now the bay had an inlet almost directly south of the Shinnecock Canal (opened more than 40 years prior) that would save boats a trip of many miles to access the ocean. The cut was stabilized, docks were built, and in a few years a small fleet of fishing vessels settled in to call Shinnecock home. Amazingly, little has changed since.

Even though Shinnecock Bay is not especially large—it stretches roughly 8 miles west to east, from Quogue to Southampton—it packs an incredible number of sights and natural features along its shores. Its easternmost barrier beach is replete with immense oceanfront mansions and some smaller bayside bungalows, many of which are almost too beautiful to believe. The barrier beach to the west is totally different, with nothing more than salt marsh and a few small parking areas for surfers and beachgoers. Many more houses sit along Shinnecock's northern shore, in equally high numbers on either side of the Ponquogue Bridge that separates the bay into an eastern and western half. Plus, a few sandy islands sit just above the inlet, the canal leading to Peconic Bay opens to the north, and the historic Shinnecock Indian Reservation makes up a good portion of the bay's easternmost shore.

Despite Shinnecock Bay's relatively small size, paddling from one side to the other may be too long a trip for many paddlers. Luckily, a multitude of put-ins circle the bay, making such a trip unnecessary. Anyone with a Southampton municipal permit can park at any of the various turnoffs on Dune Road and Meadow Lane, and parking at Shinnecock East County Park, on the inlet's east side, requires only a small fee. Otherwise, the parking area at the southern base of the Ponquogue Bridge is open to anyone, as is the one at the end of Ox Pasture Road in the village of Southampton. My usual put-in is off Little Neck Road on Old Fort Pond, where a dirt lot and small beach welcome all paddlers.

USGS Quadrangles
SOUTHAMPTON (NY),
SHINNECOCK INLET (NY)

32 **DESCRIPTION** Launching from the small beach off Little Neck Road puts you on a small section of Shinnecock Bay known as Old Fort Pond. I've long felt a strong affection for this tiny body of water, having spent much of my undergraduate career at the Marine Station at Southampton College (now part of Stony Brook University), near its northern end. Because of its proximity to both the Shinnecock Canal and Shinnecock Inlet, Old Fort

Old Fort Pond to Meadow Lane and Back

Level	2B
Distance	8.6 miles round-trip
Time	3 hours
Navigable months	Year-round
Hazards	Open water
Portages	None
Rescue access	Easy
Tidal conditions	3 hours before or after high tide
Scenery	A

Pond is the ideal site for such a facility, as well as a marina or two. Paddle beside its shore and you'll pass these two marinas, the marine station, and a number of waterfront homes along the way. In fact, most of the pond's western and northern shores are filled with one type of structure or another. Cross to its eastern side though, and you'll be greeted by a shoreline almost completely devoid of development.

Along this side of Old Fort Pond lies the Shinnecock Indian Reservation. Comprising almost 1,200 acres, the reservation is home to more than 600 nationally recognized members of the Shinnecock Nation, one of the oldest self-governing Native American tribes in the country. Its members have constructed a health-care center, a church, an education center, playgrounds, and a museum on the reservation and have also successfully run a shellfish hatchery for many years; little, if any, of this is visible from the seat of a kayak, however. Instead, a sandy beach leading up to a narrow band of spartina grass and dense woodland beyond makes up the majority of the scene.

Continue paddling south along the reservation's shore and you'll reach a small cove directly opposite your put-in. If you look to the pebble-strewn spit of land separating it from the bay, you may catch a glimpse of some of Shinnecock's common summer residents: least terns. Easily identified by their white, streamlined bodies, black heads, and yellow beaks and legs, these birds are often seen diving headfirst into the water to catch a fish. They also tend to congregate along this stretch of shoreline, so keep an eye out for any that happen to be land-bound.

You'll be able to hug the reservation's unbroken shoreline for most of the next mile as you head south, although the water may be too shallow in spots to float a kayak, thus forcing you to alter your course a bit. If the tide is too low for you to paddle close to shore, it certainly won't be conducive for paddling into the small pond near the reservation's southern tip. In fact, it may even be too shallow to allow you easy passage to the reservation's eastern shore. Examine the area using Google Earth, and you'll see

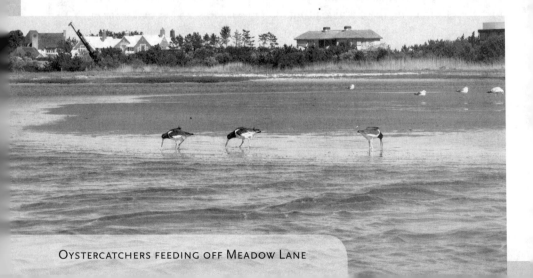

Oystercatchers feeding off Meadow Lane

just how extensive the shoal in this section of Shinnecock Bay is. Luckily, we kayakers need only get out of our boats and wade a bit to find water deep enough for our shallow-draft boats.

Once you've rounded the peninsula, turn your bow to the north and Heady Creek will lie dead ahead. Mostly developed and fairly shallow, this creek stretches almost 1.5 miles to the north, then ends just a few hundred feet before it reaches Montauk Highway. While it contains little in the way of natural beauty, Heady Creek does have an excellent put-in site, at the end of Ox Pasture Road.

As you paddle out of Heady Creek and begin to turn east toward Taylor Creek, the Ruth Wales DuPont Sanctuary lies just off your boat to the left. Consisting of 32 acres of lush salt marsh, the preserve is home to an active osprey nest as well as numerous wading birds, such as snowy egrets, willets, and lesser yellowlegs. The DuPont family purchased the land that the preserve sits on long ago so they would have an undisturbed view from their mansion across the water on Meadow Lane. It was this same desire to protect the land as open space that helped create the preserve we know today.

Now that you're along the southern shore of Shinnecock Bay, stay close to

the water's edge and you'll marvel at the many oceanfront mansions lining the south side of Southampton's Meadow Lane. You'll also be able to paddle beside the lush salt marsh that borders its northern side. Continue in this direction about 3 miles and you'll reach the Shinnecock Inlet, the Ponquogue Bridge, and the western portion of the bay. Along the way you'll float past dozens of channels, cuts, and coves in the marsh that hide beautiful species of birds, from great blue herons to great egrets, oystercatchers to ospreys. It's not a stretch of the imagination to say that this section of water is a veritable sea kayaker's paradise.

As you paddle along this remarkable stretch of land and water, remember that you still have to cross the bay to get back to Old Fort Pond and your take-out. You don't want to travel too far or risk being faced with a crossing longer than you would like (for example, the distance from the inlet to Old Fort Pond is 3 miles). So enjoy the paddling and revel in the view, but reserve some time and energy for that paddle back across Shinnecock Bay.

✧ **SHUTTLE DIRECTIONS** To get to the put-in on Little Neck Road, take Sunrise Highway (NY 27) to the Shinnecock Hills portion of Southampton. Turn right (left if coming from the east) onto Tuckahoe Road at the sign for the Stony Brook University Southampton Campus, and travel south 0.4 mile. Cross over Montauk Highway (NY 27A) and continue south on Little Neck Road 0.6 mile. Look for the dirt lot and small beach on the left side of Little Neck Road.

GPS COORDINATES

Put-in/take-out
N40° 52.655' W72° 26.566'
Tide station
Ponquogue Bridge,
Shinnecock Bay, NY
N40° 51.000' W72° 30.000'

33 STONY BROOK HARBOR

✧ **OVERVIEW** Stony Brook Harbor, along the North Shore of Long Island, provides paddlers with an amazingly beautiful tidal estuary to explore. This is one of my favorite places to paddle: the area is rich in history, the scenery is exquisite, the water is almost always calm, and the wildlife is plentiful. If you seek a place to spend a few hours or pass an entire day, Stony Brook Harbor has what you're looking for.

Before you head out on a paddle here, always remember to check the tides. Many parts of the harbor become little more than mudflats during low tide. In addition, currents near the northern end of the harbor can move quite swiftly during tidal changes. For the best conditions, time your departure so you can ride the incoming tide to the back of the harbor. Then stay

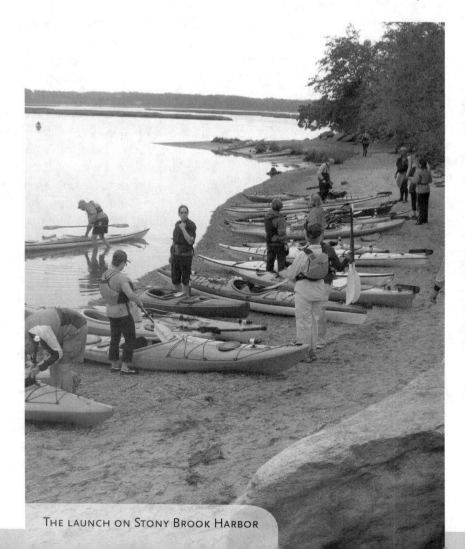

THE LAUNCH ON STONY BROOK HARBOR

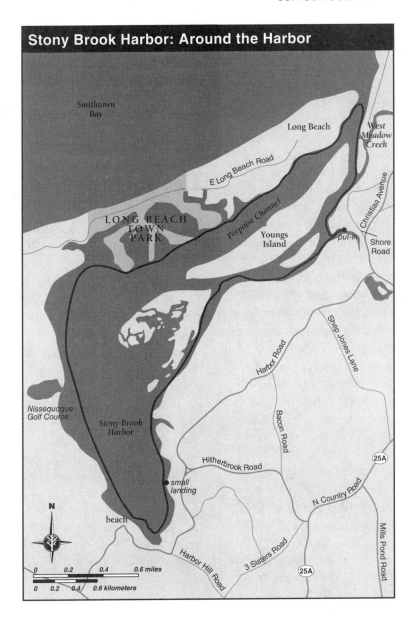

Stony Brook Harbor: Around the Harbor

Smithtown Bay

Long Beach

West Meadow Creek

E Long Beach Road

Christian Avenue

LONG BEACH TOWN PARK

Porpoise Channel

Youngs Island

put-in

Shore Road

Nissequogue Golf Course

Stony Brook Harbor

Shep Jones Lane

Harbor Road

Bacon Road

Hitherbrook Road

25A

small landing

N

beach

N Country Road

3 Sisters Road

25A

Mills Pond Road

Harbor Hill Road

0   0.2   0.4   0.6 miles

0   0.2   0.4   0.6 kilometers

long enough for the tide to change—quite easy to do in a place as appealing as Stony Brook—and follow the outgoing tide back to your launch site.

But be sure to watch for the amazing variety of wildlife that calls Stony Brook Harbor home. Bird-watchers will marvel at the incredible numbers of great blue herons, great and snowy egrets, black-crowned night herons, least terns, and American oystercatchers, while fishermen will appreciate the large schools of bluefish and striped bass. I've even witnessed congregations of well over 100 diamondback terrapin turtles poking their little heads just above the water's surface here. Add an 18th-century gristmill, a 19th-century shipbuilding legacy, and enough charm to warm anyone's soul, and it's easy to understand Stony Brook Harbor's draw.

The best place to launch is at the small beach next to the parking lot of the Three Village Inn. It provides free parking year-round for both residents and nonresidents, unlike the nearby town boat ramp, which charges for daily and seasonal use. Or you can launch off Sand Street Beach, a bit farther north of the boat ramp. This is a useful option during low tides when there's not enough water by the parking lot, although it does require a bit more work—you'll have to drop off your gear by the beach's bathhouse, park your car in the nearby lot, and carry your boat the short distance from the bathhouse to the water.

Should you choose to venture out of Stony Brook Harbor into Smithtown Bay, you can extend your trip by heading northeast to West Meadow Beach, a fairly large beach with bathrooms, water fountains, and usually an ice-cream truck or two. From there you can continue your adventure by heading north to the point of land known as Crane's Neck, where you can paddle and play among many large boulders, or erratics, that were deposited by a glacier more than 10,000 years ago. Use your imagination and pretend you're paddling off the rocky coast of Maine. If Crane's Neck seems too far and West Meadow Beach is too crowded, try paddling West Meadow Creek (see page 171) instead. You won't be disappointed.

USGS Quadrangles
SAINT JAMES (NY)

Mean Water Temperatures by Month (°F)					
	JAN	FEB	MAR	APR	MAY	JUN
MEAN	37	36	39	46	55	63
	JUL	AUG	SEP	OCT	NOV	DEC
MEAN	70	73	70	61	50	41

33 **DESCRIPTION** Launching from the small beach off the town parking lot positions you optimally to begin a trip deep into the harbor itself. Paddling straight off the beach brings you to a fairly large piece of land, known as Young's Island, that's worthy of a circumnavigation. Resist the urge to land there, however, as the entire island is a designated bird sanctuary. Regardless, you can see an amazing variety of birds from the water.

Paddle here during the spring and summer, and you'll surely encounter the tiny yet bold least tern. Individuals from their large colony can usually be seen flying about the harbor, emitting their short *kip-kip-kip* calls. Watch them scout for small fish from the air and dive-bomb the water to snag a quick meal. While the large numbers of terns around the harbor seem to indicate a healthy population, these birds are actually endangered. So give them a wide berth, especially when they are nesting. Continue south around Young's Island and you will likely see another beautiful bird, the great blue heron. If you do, it may be a sight you'll never forget: with its imposing stature (great blue herons can stand 4 feet tall) and striking blue-and-gray plumage, the bird has a way of etching itself into your memory.

Around the Harbor

Level	2B
Distance	7 miles around
Time	4 hours
Navigable months	Year-round
Hazards	Boat traffic, tidal currents
Portages	None
Rescue access	Easy
Tidal conditions	3 hours before or after high tide
Scenery	A+

Southwest of Young's Island lie large mussel banks and low-lying spartina-grass islands, with a maze of large and small channels in between. Some are paddle-friendly, others are not. Dead ends, wrong turns, and vast mudflats can make paddling through this section an enjoyable yet slightly adventurous part of your trip. I always make it a point to explore this part of the harbor whenever I have the chance.

Continue south for another mile and you'll enter a large expanse of water as the harbor widens. By this point, you may have already noticed that although the shore is dotted with some beautiful waterfront homes, the harbor has a pristine feel to it. In fact, most of the buildings surrounding it are hidden behind vast stands of locust, oak, and beech, making it quite easy to forget they are there at all. While most of these houses have private beaches complete with the requisite NO TRESPASSING signs, two tiny yet welcoming beaches are just 2 and 2.5 miles, respectively, after the put-in

if you need to land and stretch your legs. Both beaches also provide limited parking and can be used as alternative launching points.

After resting a bit on either beach or exploring the freshwater creek that empties into the harbor in its southeast corner, you can follow the eastern shore back to your starting point or follow the western shore of the harbor as it curves north. There is much to see on this side of the harbor, including a small pond centered in a golf course and a Town of Smithtown park called Long Beach. The entrance to the pond is just 0.8 mile north of the southernmost beach, under the wooden bridge visible from the harbor. Remember, though, that paddling the pond is tide-dependent and can be quite dangerous (depending on the skill levels of the golfers, of course).

Three-quarters of a mile to the north lies a mooring field, with Long Beach to the west. Many bird boxes and an active osprey platform are here. Young's Island is just 1 mile farther north, with a stretch of water called Porpoise Channel connecting the harbor to Smithtown Bay beyond that. Paddling around Young's Island and through Porpoise Channel is trouble-free as long as you are paddling with the tide. Currents here can quickly become swift and dangerous, however, and should only

GPS COORDINATES

Put-in/take-out
N40° 55.122' W73° 09.023'
Tide station
Stony Brook, Smithtown Bay, NY
N400 55.002' W730 09.000'

be paddled under ideal conditions. (The alternative may find you paddling furiously against both tide and boat traffic, fighting to make the slightest headway.) A safer option, when water levels are high enough, is to cut through the marsh south of Young's Island and bypass Porpoise Channel altogether. From there, your put-in is only a short paddle away.

✧ **SHUTTLE DIRECTIONS** To get to the launch site in Stony Brook Village, take the Long Island Expressway (I-495) east to Exit 62 (Nichols Road/CR-97) and follow the signs north to Stony Brook. CR-97 will continue 11 miles before ending at a stoplight. At this point, turn left onto SR 25A. Head west 1 mile, taking the right fork onto Main Street. You will reach the Three Village Inn after 0.5 mile. Go straight around the traffic circle and continue on to Shore Road. The parking lot and small beach will be on your left before the boat marina.

34 SWAN RIVER

✧ **OVERVIEW** One of only a few spring-fed streams on Long Island that are still free-flowing, the Swan River, in the South Shore town of Patchogue, may be the cleanest and most unspoiled of them all. It begins as a diminutive freshwater spring south of the Long Island Expressway, picking up a bit of speed and growing in size until it flows into Patchogue's Swan Lake, just north of Montauk Highway. The river then becomes tidal below the lake, forming a brackish estuary before it empties into Patchogue Bay and the Great South Bay. Considering the densely populated neighborhoods the river flows through, it's quite remarkable that much of the Swan's shoreline has escaped development, remaining mostly forested wetland to this day.

Since the Native Americans inhabited the area hundreds of years ago, Patchogue and portions of the Swan River have been an important source of both finfish and shellfish. Seventeenth-century English settlers used the land in much the same way, helping foster the birth of an industry that is still alive today, albeit on a much smaller scale. Shellfish, especially oysters, were famously harvested from the waters around Patchogue and, as the business grew, were sold to markets and restaurants worldwide. In fact, this is where the term "Blue Point Oyster" originated. Unfortunately, most of the trade has diminished, although a few baymen still work the waters off the Swan River and the Great South Bay in search of the bivalve.

While oysters are very hard to come by these days, the clean, fresh water of the Swan River's upper portion nurtures brook trout (the river contains one of only six wild populations of the fish found on the island), while the lower, tidal segment of the river is ideal for spawning brown trout. Juvenile bluefish, wading shorebirds, and many species of waterfowl also make a claim to the Swan's waters.

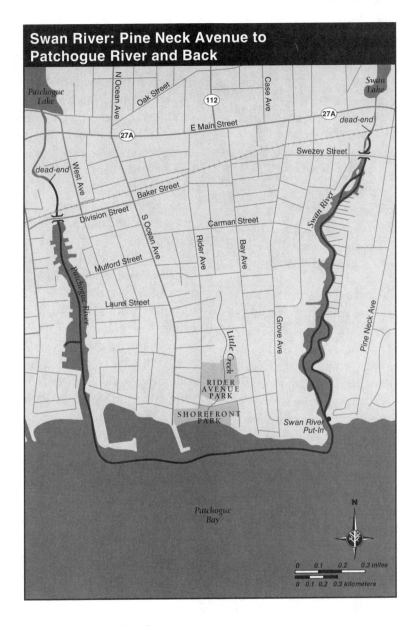

Swan River: Pine Neck Avenue to Patchogue River and Back

Those wanting to paddle along the river and experience its natural beauty for themselves can find no better put-in than at the end of Pine Neck Avenue. Anyone may use the small boat ramp found there; parking is free. The site is open only from sunrise to sunset, however, so plan your trip accordingly.

USGS Quadrangles Howells Point (NY), Bellport (NY), Sayville (NY), Patchogue (NY)

34 DESCRIPTION Although the Great South Bay beckons just a few hundred feet south of the put-in, heading north on the Swan River provides paddlers with a surprisingly scenic

Pine Neck Avenue to Patchogue River and Back

Level	2B
Distance	7.5 miles round-trip
Time	3 hours
Navigable months	Year-round
Hazards	Boat traffic
Portages	None
Rescue access	Easy
Tidal conditions	Any
Scenery	C+/B

route to follow. Immediately south of the boat ramp stretches a wooden dock that is a popular crabbing and fishing spot for locals, while another dock to the north marks the site of a small marina. Just a few paddle strokes are all it takes to leave both docks behind, though, and enter a relatively unspoiled area. Both sides of the river are lined with fairly extensive salt marsh, with spartina growing at the water's edge, followed by phragmites in some spots and a typical salt-marsh plant called marsh elder in other spots. Great and snowy egrets are numerous along this stretch of river, as are red-winged blackbirds and common terns. Fish like striped bass, bluefish, and brown trout also populate this estuarine portion of the Swan River.

A second marina lies on the river's left (west) bank 0.3 mile north of the put-in, with another appearing shortly after, and a handful of houses 0.25 mile later. The right-hand (east) side of the river runs unbroken for much of its length, however, with only a few houses

appearing just before the river reaches the end of its navigable portion.

Between the last few houses and the northern terminus of the river sits an extremely short, yet fascinating stretch of water that is completely different from that of the previous 1.2 miles. When the river passes under the Swezey Street Bridge, it enters a new environment where salt marsh is replaced with fresh. Gone are the spartina grasses and egrets of the lower estuary. Enter silver and red maple trees, alder bushes, water willow, and other freshwater plants. Paddling under the bridge is almost like stepping into a new world. Unfortunately, the feeling is very short-lived, as the river becomes impassable at the railroad trestle. There is talk of installing a fish ladder here to aid alewives in swimming upstream to spawn. Perhaps a portage from Swan River into Swan Lake, just a bit upstream, may soon be possible as well.

The navigable portion of the Swan River runs for 2.6 miles round-trip. For some paddlers, that may be enough. Others may want more, however, in which case they can make an additional trip out on the Great South Bay to another nearby river, the Patchogue. From the mouth of the Swan, the Patchogue is just 1 mile west, along the bay's northern shore.

GPS COORDINATES

Put-in/take-out
N40° 44.942' W72° 59.860'
Tide station
Patchogue, NY
N40° 45.498' W73° 01.200'

Look for its entrance just beyond the second pier.

A paddle up the Patchogue contrasts sharply with the Swan's relatively pristine environment. Docks, docks, and more docks float everywhere along this river. It is a true boat-watcher's paradise, for even when there are no docks, there are boatyards, yacht clubs, and marinas. There are even restaurants that cater to boats scattered throughout. Obviously, nature observation has to take a break on the Patchogue, at least on its lower stretches. But paddle up its 1-mile length, pass under a small bridge at Division Street, and as on the Swan, a different world waits.

The Patchogue becomes much narrower in this new section, lined with large maple and catalpa trees that block out most of the sun. Alder bushes abound here, as do Japanese knotweed,

wild grape, and water willow. I was even lucky enough to glimpse a few black-crowned night herons among the trees when I last paddled here. But like the Swan River, the Patchogue dead-ends all too soon, forcing you to turn around and head back the way you came, 2.5 miles back to the boat launch at the mouth of the Swan.

✧ **SHUTTLE DIRECTIONS** To get to the put-in off Pine Neck Avenue, take NY 27 (Sunrise Highway) to Exit 53S (NY 112). Head south on NY 112 until it ends at NY 27A (Montauk Highway) 0.8 mile later. Turn left onto Montauk Highway and head east 0.7 mile before turning right onto Country Road. Take your first right turn onto Pine Neck Avenue and follow it 1.3 miles south. Look for the entrance to the town boat launch at the end of the road, on the right.

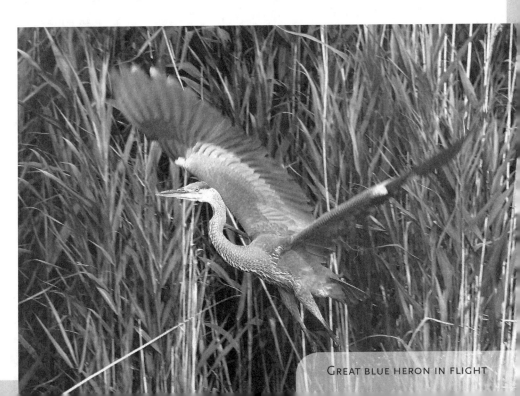

GREAT BLUE HERON IN FLIGHT

35 THREE MILE HARBOR

✧ **OVERVIEW** Three Mile Harbor is one of the most beautiful harbors on Long Island. About 3 miles north of the town of East Hampton (hence its name), the harbor is a popular destination for sailors, powerboaters, and paddlers alike. Its eastern shore, replete with marinas, can be quite busy at times, while the western shore can be most peaceful and serene. Its southern end is fairly developed, whereas its northern end is more natural with bountiful wildlife. Indeed, these contrasts help give Three Mile Harbor its personality and make it, as author Sylvia Mendelman says, "East Hampton's priceless gem."

While the marinas and their associated yachts may provide some attraction, most paddlers seek out locations with more natural beauty. If this is for you, Three Mile Harbor will not disappoint. Whether you explore the undeveloped western shore near Hands Creek or wind your way through the tidal marshes of Goose Creek, nothing but birds, fish, and lush plant life will be there to keep you company. Ospreys, egrets, and herons are quite common, while American oystercatchers, black-bellied plovers, and other wading birds make frequent guest appearances. Bluefish and striped bass are common in the harbor's waters, as are diamondback terrapins and all the usual crustaceans. Spartina marshes line the shores, stately trees pepper the landscape, and waves lap the pebble beaches. Three Mile Harbor truly is a paddler's delight.

Three Mile Harbor presents paddlers with one small problem, however: parking. You'll find a number of convenient launch spots around the harbor; unfortunately, most of them require a town permit to park. While some of the marinas may sometimes let paddlers launch boats from their docks or ramps, the best put-in I've found—one that's free, public, and safe to use—is at the end of a dead-end road called Will Curl Highway.

USGS Quadrangles
GARDINERS ISLAND WEST (NY), EAST HAMPTON (NY)

35 **DESCRIPTION** Launching from the small, rocky beach at the end of Will Curl Highway puts the entire harbor in front of you. Head south and you'll be paddling alongside dozens of waterfront homes for the next 0.5 mile, after which you reach the

Around the Harbor

Level	2B
Distance	7 miles around
Time	4 hours
Navigable months	Year-round
Hazards	Boat traffic
Portages	None
Rescue access	Easy
Tidal conditions	4 hours before or after high tide
Scenery	A+

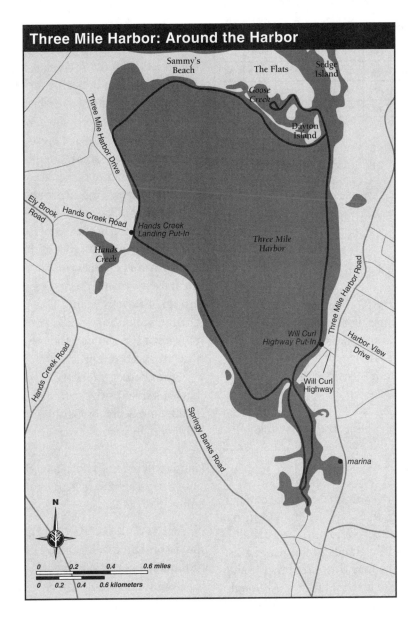

Three Mile Harbor: Around the Harbor

GPS COORDINATES

Put-in/take-out
N41° 00.633' W72° 10.980'
Tide station
Three Mile Harbor Entrance,
Gardiners Bay, NY
N41° 02.100' W72° 11.400'

southernmost portion of the harbor and its sprawling marinas. Of course, with marinas come powerboats, so take care when paddling here, especially in the summer.

A small creek flows into the harbor 1 mile south of the launch site. Navigable during high tide only, this

Mean Water Temperatures by Month (°F)					
	JAN	FEB	MAR	APR	MAY	JUN
MEAN	36	37	39	46	53	64
	JUL	AUG	SEP	OCT	NOV	DEC
MEAN	72	77	72	65	52	41

creek does extend south far enough to warrant exploration if time allows. If not, the large coves to the west are quite paddle-friendly. From here, the only direction to paddle is north, toward the vast expanse of water that is Three Mile Harbor.

A small, sandy island juts out into the harbor 0.5 mile to the north. Like most of the land lining this part of the harbor, this island is marked PRIVATE and landing is forbidden. Its beauty, and its resident osprey, are easily visible from the water, though, and make for great photo ops. Little else but houses can be seen along the next mile of shoreline, until it is broken by a wide swath of wooded land and a small section of water called Hands Creek. While not very large, the creek does provide an additional 0.5 mile or so of paddling, with a convenient put-in spot (Hands Creek Landing) immediately to the north. Hands Creek also marks the point where the more pristine side of the harbor starts to show. Although houses stand along the shoreline north of here, they are fairly well hidden behind large oaks and other trees, almost disappearing altogether.

Sammy's Beach, just 1 mile north of the creek, marks the northernmost border of the harbor. It also contains a hidden gem on its eastern end: Goose Creek. A tidal waterway with two inlets, one at either end, this creek is a paddling destination in itself. It shelters an amazing variety of shorebirds, from oystercatchers, willets, dowitchers, and plovers to terns, egrets, herons, and dunlins. Ospreys are frequently seen here, as are diamondback terrapins, horseshoe crabs, and many species of fish. Look for Goose Creek's western entrance on the harbor side of Sammy's Beach, just a bit east of the osprey platform, and its eastern entrance near the harbor's inlet, around the northern tip of Dayton Island. This maze of channels and dead ends is accessible only during high tides, though, so plan your trip accordingly.

From here, a short paddle out the harbor's inlet brings you to either Maidstone Beach or Gardiners Bay, both equally attractive destinations. Alternately, paddling 1.5 miles to the south will bring you back to your put-in—a good spot to rest after a long but enjoyable paddle.

✧ **SHUTTLE DIRECTIONS** To get to the put-in on Three Mile Harbor, take SR 27 (Montauk Highway) into East Hampton. Continue through town on SR 27 until North Main Street branches off just south of the large windmill. Head north on North Main Street (it will turn into Three Mile Harbor Road) for 3.1 miles and turn left onto Will Curl Highway. Park at the end of the road and follow the short path to the beach.

36 WEST MEADOW CREEK

✧ **OVERVIEW** Though its small size has kept it from becoming widely known among the paddling community, West Meadow Creek is one of Long Island's true hidden treasures— a treat for all who visit it. It's tucked away within an almost 100-acre-wide salt marsh just north of Stony Brook Harbor, flowing north to south for about 2 miles before it empties into Smithtown Bay. Along the way, it passes a historic horse farm, dozens of picturesque Colonial-era homes, and little else besides the lush, verdant marsh spoken of earlier. In fact, the natural beauty of the creek and the environment it flows through are its biggest draws.

Amazingly, West Meadow Creek was not always as scenic as it is now. In fact, the entire peninsula that separates the creek from Smithtown Bay

was once lined with beach cottages and summer houses. Hardly more than rustic shacks constructed in the 1920s and 1930s, many had been passed down through families for years. But a fierce debate sprang up in 1996, as New York State sought to protect its open spaces and threatened to evict the cottages' residents (the buildings had been constructed on state land). Cottage owners and locals on their side fought the government in a campaign they called Save the Cottages, mainly citing family ties and a historic designation as their reasons for staying. Unfortunately for them, the state did tear down all but a very few of the buildings in 2004. Luckily for the public, what was left was a paved road for walkers, bikers, and joggers, benches for resting and picnicking, and undisturbed water views almost every way you look. As for paddlers, an undeveloped shore lined with red cedar trees and spartina grass was our gift.

If you want to experience this amazing place for yourself, the best

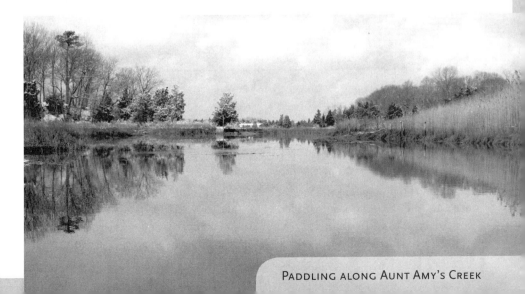

PADDLING ALONG AUNT AMY'S CREEK

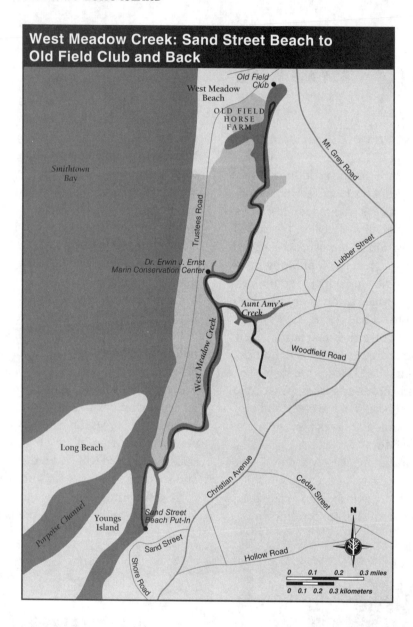

West Meadow Creek: Sand Street Beach to Old Field Club and Back

put-in spot is Sand Street Beach in Stony Brook. From its shore you'll have two options for gaining access to the creek. The first entails paddling a short distance along Porpoise Channel until you've rounded a small island marking the creek's southern border, though boat traffic and strong tidal currents (especially during a flood tide) can sometimes make this stretch quite a challenge. The second option—hugging the beach and paddling between it and the small island—is much easier and safer. Unfortunately, there isn't always enough water to accomplish this. In that case, your best bet is to launch near the end of the incoming tide so you can ride its current up the creek, then easily return as the tide ebbs.

USGS Quadrangles
SAINT JAMES (NY)

36 **DESCRIPTION** Whichever direction you come from when heading toward West Meadow Creek, the first thing you'll likely notice is the charming beach cottage at its mouth. Known locally as the Gamecock Cottage, this green-and-red building was built in the mid-1800s as an aviary. It originally sat on land much higher and drier than now, almost 0.5 mile away. Since being moved to its current location, the cottage has been used as both a boathouse and a summer rental. Luckily, it has been kept in excellent condition and has become an iconic landmark for all to enjoy.

Look across to the opposite side of the creek as you pass the Gamecock Cottage, and you'll find another interesting sight: a life-size statue of a pirate standing watch over the water. More than once I've tricked a paddling companion into thinking it was a real person watching us kayak by.

Many more houses pop up beyond the pirate, although they're built a bit higher up the steep bluff that lines the creek's right-hand (eastern) shoreline. Without gazing upwards, you would know they were there only because of the flights of wooden stairs that run from their properties to the water's edge. The welcome effect is that it's almost possible to forget the houses even exist. The left (west) side of the creek is completely

Sand Street Beach to Old Field Club and Back

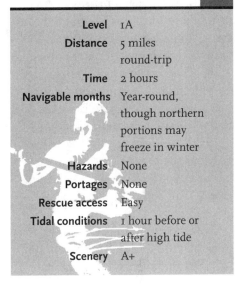

Level	1A
Distance	5 miles round-trip
Time	2 hours
Navigable months	Year-round, though northern portions may freeze in winter
Hazards	None
Portages	None
Rescue access	Easy
Tidal conditions	1 hour before or after high tide
Scenery	A+

undeveloped, adding to the beauty of the surroundings.

The creek takes a sharp right turn just 0.2 mile beyond the Gamecock Cottage, followed by a quick left that will have you heading north once again. Look to the left (west) as you continue paddling upstream, and you should get a sense of how vast the salt marsh along the creek is. See the red cedar trees in the distance? Everything between them and you is marsh, with spartina (smooth cordgrass) the dominant species. Other species grow here as well,

GPS COORDINATES

Put-in/take-out
N40° 53.847' W73° 26.082'
Tide station
Stony Brook, Smithtown Bay, NY
N40° 55.002' W73° 09.000'

albeit a bit higher up on drier land. Marsh elder, bayberry, the infamous poison ivy, and even prickly pear cacti grow along the creek's borders. From the seat of a kayak, though, only the grasses that enjoy a frequent dousing with salt water are easily visible.

The creek then runs almost due north for the next 0.5 mile, with marsh to the left and oak- and maple-lined bluffs to the right. If you look to the right just before the creek begins a lazy left turn, you'll see where a small side creek, Aunt Amy's Creek, branches off the main flow. With a mile of shoreline of its own, Aunt Amy's Creek is a great place to explore should you have the time and energy. It has its share of houses and docks, most of which are built quite close together and right on the water, but it also has its share of scenic views and photo spots.

If you opt to paddle Aunt Amy's Creek, you'll notice that it divides into two distinct arms just a few hundred feet from its entrance. Though they're equal in distance, the southern arm has a bit of an advantage over the northern arm in that it contains a small marshy area, whereas the northern arm consists of mostly developed shoreline. Still, it's just as enjoyable to paddle as its less-developed counterpart.

As you leave the side creek and continue north, West Meadow Creek turns almost 180 degrees to the east. At the apex of the curve sits the Dr. Erwin J. Ernst Marine Conservation Center. Named after a beloved local teacher, it hosts lectures, classes, guided hikes, and summer camps, all of which are designed to educate the public about

the amazing ecosystem they live in. I was lucky enough to have Dr. Ernst as a professor years ago, and I'm sure he'd be honored to see the work being done in his name.

While you may not be able to take advantage of the conservation center's educational programs while paddling, you can make great use of a unique feature on its property. Land your boat on the beach below the center and walk to the opposite side of the building. There you'll find a small metal pipe coming out of the ground, flowing with water. Take a deep drink from this natural spring and top off your water bottle before you return to the creek. Coming straight from Long Island's aquifer system, the water could not be more crisp or clean.

Once you've quenched your thirst and relaunched your kayak, continue paddling upstream and you'll come to a section of marsh that is significantly more vast than that downstream. It continues another 0.3 mile before you skirt around a small private beach club on the opposite shore. Paddle past its swing sets, pavilion, and kayak racks, and you'll come to a small cove that borders a portion of the Old Field Horse Farm.

West Meadow Creek comes to an end just a few hundred feet upstream of the horse farm, although there's one more item of interest to see before you turn around. Another historic building, this one housing the Old Field Club, sits on the western bank just before the creek dead-ends. Built in 1929, it was originally a bathing club, then a beach and tennis club. It now functions as an elegant catering hall where many private parties and weddings take place each year. With any luck, such an event will be taking place as you paddle by, and you may just end up in someone's wedding photos.

Not much is left to see on West Meadow Creek once you've passed the Old Field Club. Simply turn your kayak around, start paddling downstream, and enjoy all of the creek's scenery once again. You'll have 2 miles to do so.

✧ **SHUTTLE DIRECTIONS** To get to the put-in at Sand Street Beach, take the Long Island Expressway (I-495) east to Exit 62 (Nichols Road/CR-97) and follow the signs north to Stony Brook. CR-97 continues 11 miles before it ends at a stoplight. At this point, turn left onto NY 25A. Head west 1 mile before taking the right fork onto Main Street. You'll reach the Three Village Inn after 0.5 mile. Go straight around the traffic circle and continue on to Shore Road. You'll pass a marina and yacht club before coming to the pavilion at Sand Street Beach. Drop off your boat and gear there, but park by the yacht club.

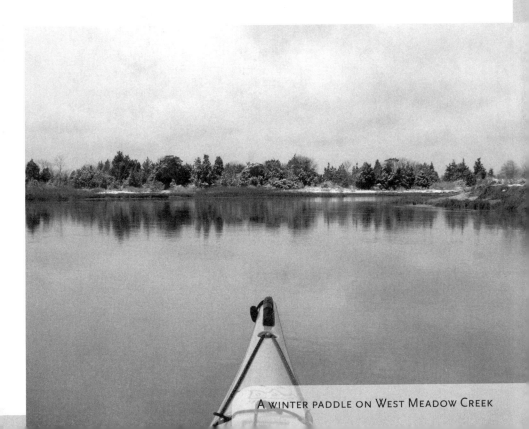

A WINTER PADDLE ON WEST MEADOW CREEK

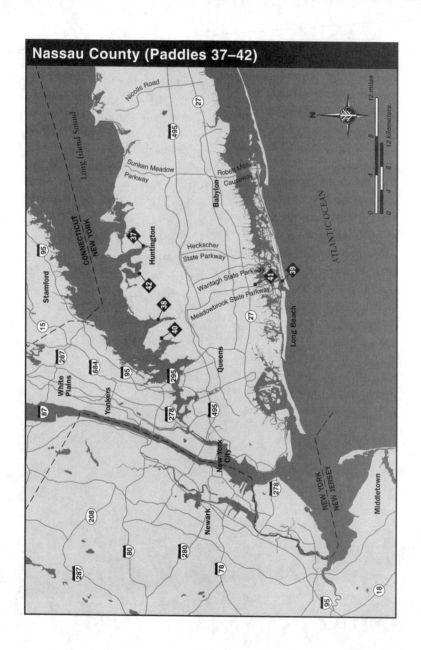

Nassau County (Paddles 37–42)

Nicolls Road

27

495

Long Island Sound

Sunken Meadow
Parkway

Robert Moses
Causeway

Babylon

CONNECTICUT
NEW YORK

95

Stamford

37

Huntington

Heckscher
State Parkway

42

38

Wantagh State Parkway

39

41

15

Meadowbrook State Parkway

287

40

Long Beach

ATLANTIC OCEAN

684

95

White
Plains

Yonkers

95

295

27

Queens

87

278

495

New York
City

278

New York
New Jersey

Middletown

208

Newark

280

80

287

78

95

18

N

12 miles

12 kilometers

8

4

8

4

8

0

0

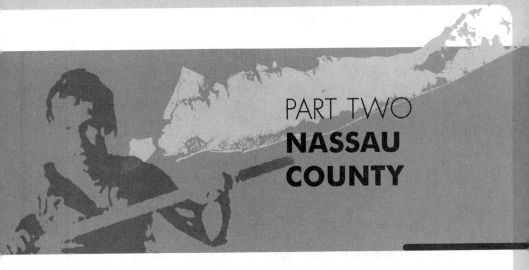

37 COLD SPRING HARBOR

◇ **OVERVIEW** Nestled between Oyster Bay and Huntington harbors, on Long Island's affluent North Shore, Cold Spring Harbor is a fairly large body of water steeped in maritime history. It was the Native Americans who originally recognized the area's value as a source of game, finfish and shellfish, and fresh water. They called it *Wawapeck,* or "The Little Place with Good Water," in reference to the freshwater springs. Although the colonizing Europeans eventually changed the harbor's name, the importance of the springs was not lost to them. As a result, they chose "Cold Spring" to describe it.

The Europeans were also quick to appreciate the fertility of the land, its plentiful wildlife, and its deep and protected harbor. Milling, fishing, and shipbuilding became important businesses in the area during the 17th and 18th centuries. Not until the 19th century, though, did the harbor reach its prominence as an East Coast whaling port. In fact, by the middle of that century, it supported a fleet of nine large whaling ships. Of course, there were other ports much bigger and more successful than Cold Spring Harbor; nevertheless, the whaling industry was the lifeblood of the town and helped solidify its presence on the map.

With the end of whaling in the late 19th century, Cold Spring Harbor shifted its focus from bustling port to resort town. Hotels and restaurants opened, and the town began catering to vacationers looking to escape New York City. Then, in 1890, a new venture came to the area: a laboratory was built on land once owned by the Cold Spring Whaling Company, and classes were started to train high school and college teachers in marine biology. The lab, originally an extension of the Brooklyn Institute of Arts and Sciences and later named Cold Spring Harbor Laboratory, began to expand its courses of study to include the growing field of genetics. Fast-forward to

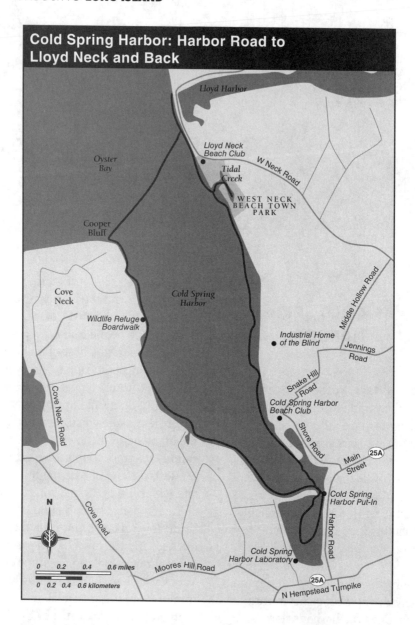

Cold Spring Harbor: Harbor Road to Lloyd Neck and Back

Lloyd Harbor

Lloyd Neck
Beach Club

*Oyster
Bay*

W Neck Road

*Tidal
Creek*

WEST NECK
BEACH TOWN
PARK

*Cooper
Bluff*

Middle Hollow Road

*Cove
Neck*

*Cold Spring
Harbor*

Wildlife Refuge
Boardwalk

Industrial Home
of the Blind

Jennings
Road

Cove Neck Road

Snake Hill
Road

Cold Spring Harbor
Beach Club

Shore Road

Main
Street

25A

N

Cold Spring
Harbor Put-In

Cove Road

Harbor Road

0   0.2   0.4   0.6 miles

Cold Spring
Harbor Laboratory

0   0.2 0.4 0.6 kilometers

Moores Hill Road

25A

N Hempstead Turnpike

1953, when the lab became the site of one of the greatest breakthroughs in biology: James Watson's and Francis Crick's discovery of the structure of DNA. Amazing scientific work continues here to this day.

The town entered the public spotlight once again in 1971, though not because of whaling or science: a relatively unknown musician named Billy Joel released his first solo album, *Cold Spring Harbor*. As the album and the singer grew in popularity, so did the town. Of course, Billy Joel can't take all of the credit for making Cold Spring Harbor what it is today. But one can argue that he did help a bit.

Forty years later, Cold Spring Harbor is as popular as ever. Charming shops and restaurants line its main street, sailboats float on its waters, and a whaling museum helps keep its maritime history alive. Scores of people visit the town every day. As kayakers, though, we can see it from its best angle: on the water. To get there, launch from the town boat ramp on Harbor Road.

USGS Quadrangles
HUNTINGTON (NY),
LLOYD HARBOR (NY)

37 **DESCRIPTION** Launching from the town boat ramp puts you in just the right position to paddle north along Cold Spring Harbor's eastern shore. But you have another option: directly across from the ramp sits Cold Spring Beach, a long, narrow strip of land that almost cuts off the southernmost part of the harbor from the rest. No paddle here would be complete without first taking at least a quick tour around this small but protected part of the harbor.

There's quite a lot of scenery packed within the beach's 1 mile of shoreline. A good number of boats moor here during boating season, with a few larger models docking midway down the eastern shore. Charming houses dating back to whaling days overlook this same shore, giving you a window into what life was like on the water during the 18th and 19th centuries. A sign of modern times sits on the opposite shore: Cold Spring Harbor Laboratory. Much of the lab is visible from the water, the most remarkable portion of which comprises three or four castlelike buildings atop a low

Harbor Road to Lloyd Neck and Back

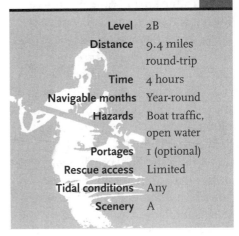

Level	2B
Distance	9.4 miles round-trip
Time	4 hours
Navigable months	Year-round
Hazards	Boat traffic, open water
Portages	1 (optional)
Rescue access	Limited
Tidal conditions	Any
Scenery	A

hill. Their colors stand out in beautiful contrast to the greens of the trees nearby. Finally, the southern side of Cold Spring Beach marks the northern boundary of this small portion of the harbor. Somewhat marshy, this piece of land is a great spot for observing birds such as egrets, terns, and black skimmers.

Kayaking through the back harbor takes only 20 minutes or so, after which you'll surely be ready to hit the main part of the harbor. Heading north along the back harbor's eastern shore lets you do just that. Just a few hundred feet north of the tip of Cold Spring Beach sits a low-lying, sandy island that can be paddled around on either side. If you need a break, it also

GPS COORDINATES

Put-in/take-out
N400 52.041' W730 27.741'
Tide station
Cold Spring Harbor, NY
N40° 52.398' W73° 28.200'

serves as a welcome rest spot, perfect for a quick snack and a drink of water. Just past the small island sits the Cold Spring Harbor Yacht Club, with a few dozen boats floating off its beach. Beyond that, there is little else in the way of unnatural distractions, with only the sound of the waves lapping on the shores and the sight of tree-lined bluffs rising up from the water's edge to keep you company.

Cold Spring Harbor has a wide (1-mile) mouth that empties into Long Island Sound between Centre Island and Lloyd Neck. On clear days, the openness of the harbor becomes pronounced once you've traveled about 1.5 miles north of your put-in. At this point you can gaze past the harbor's boundaries and see the wide expanse

of water beyond. The decks of ocean-going vessels afford bigger views, of course, but this scene is nonetheless impressive from the seat of a kayak.

The eastern shore continues uninterrupted for the next 2 miles, after which a small break in the shoreline offers an interesting side trip. Immediately after you pass a small town park on the waterfront, this break leads to a small tidal creek that in turn leads to a beautiful body of water encircled by salt marsh. Depending on the tide, the currents in the creek may be difficult to paddle against, but the view is worth the effort. On quiet days, you can sneak up on great blue herons, great egrets, and any number of other shorebirds or animals. You usually can't sneak up on the lifeguards at the

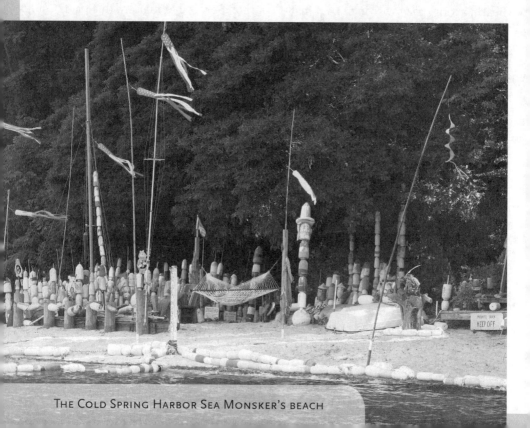

THE COLD SPRING HARBOR SEA MONSKER'S BEACH

town beach just north of the creek, though, so pass wide by the bathing area whenever swimming is in session.

The creek and town beach mark the approximate mouth of Cold Spring Harbor, although a stunning view awaits just 0.5 mile farther. Heading north and landing anywhere you can find a break in the rocky shore gives you the chance to climb up to West Neck Road and gaze down the length of the beautiful Lloyd Harbor. Intrepid kayakers may even choose to portage over the road and spend some time on that harbor's waters. Another option would be to turn around and retrace your route to its starting point. During optimal weather conditions, though, I usually opt to paddle across the harbor's mouth to Cove Neck, just 1 mile to the southwest.

Once alongside the harbor's western shore, paddlers will be sitting in the shadow of Teddy Roosevelt. His home, Sagamore Hill, sits high upon the center of the peninsula and is designated as a National Historic Site. The house is not visible from the water, but just knowing it's there is exciting.

After just a few more paddles along the western shore, kayakers will notice its relatively unspoiled nature. Much of this section of the harbor is part of the Oyster Bay National Wildlife Refuge, and thus protected from development. One of the refuge's boardwalks sits on the harbor's edge 0.5 mile south of Cove Neck's northern tip. A small creek, usually only navigable at high tide, should also be visible just

to the south of this boardwalk. The stream, which travels a short distance through a beautiful marsh in the refuge property, can provide a welcome break from the harbor's open water.

Beauty of another kind lies beyond the borders of the wildlife refuge, in the form of expansive waterfront homes that line the water's edge. In fact, little else sits on the western shore for the next 1.5 miles, although a unique site near Cold Spring Beach breaks the monotony. The home of the so-called Cold Spring Harbor Sea Monsker is replete with thousands of buoys, pieces of driftwood, flags, banners, and other assorted nautically themed items.

Such a display is a fitting way to end a trip around Cold Spring Harbor. You need only paddle a few hundred feet south from the Sea Monsker's beach to reach Cold Spring Beach. From there, the boat ramp is only a half-mile paddle away.

✧ **SHUTTLE DIRECTIONS** To get to the put-in in Cold Spring Harbor, take Interstate 495 (Long Island Expressway) to Exit 46N (Sunnyside Boulevard). Turn left onto Sunnyside Boulevard and follow it 1.1 miles to a traffic light. Turn right at the light onto Woodbury Road and take it north 3.1 miles. Turn left onto Harbor Road (NY 108) and follow it north 2.2 miles. Look for the harbor and the town boat ramp on the left side of the road. You can launch your boat here, but you may have to park in the free lot directly across the street.

38 HEMPSTEAD HARBOR

✧ **OVERVIEW** In the middle of what was once Long Island's glittering Gold Coast is a harbor that has experienced many changes in its day. Hempstead Harbor, as it has almost always been known, was the first of Long Island's harbors to be used by Europeans (Hempstead was its first colonial settlement), put into use in 1643. Those first settlers chose the area mainly because the deep, sheltered harbor was incredibly pristine and rife with natural resources. Clams, oysters, and mussels grew in abundance here, as did many species of finfish. Land containing fertile soil lined the perimeter of the harbor, and fresh-water sources were readily available. In short, Hempstead Harbor and its adjacent lands were the ideal place to settle down.

Because the harbor provided residents with almost everything they needed to survive, few felt any reason to leave. Many towns began to pop up along its shores, and with those towns came more people. And with the people came business. A mill and bustling seaport were created at the harbor's southern end in what is now Roslyn. Glen Cove also opened a mill and gained prominence as an industrial port and passenger-ship terminal. Glenwood Landing offered yet another deep-water haven for boats, and Sea Cliff, built high above the harbor's shores, earned renown as a resort town catering to the many passengers who traveled aboard the ferries that plied the harbor's waters.

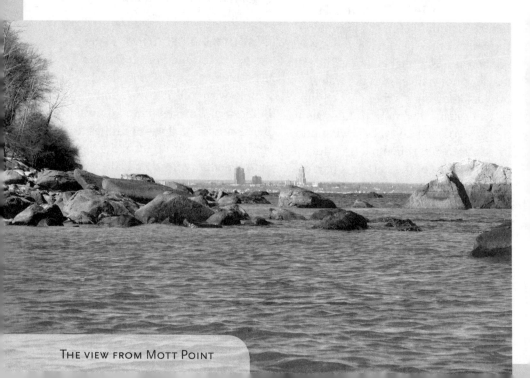

THE VIEW FROM MOTT POINT

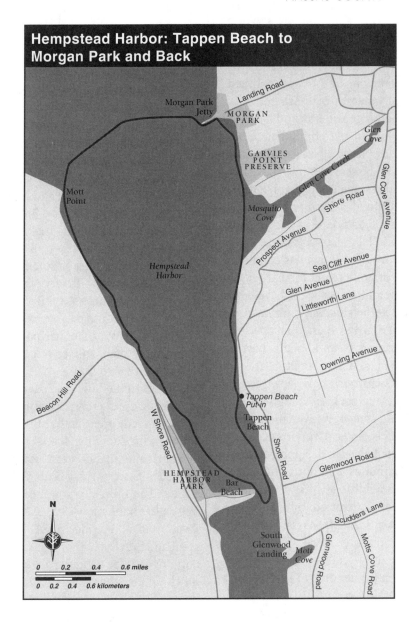

Hempstead Harbor: Tappen Beach to Morgan Park and Back

Landing Road

Morgan Park Jetty

MORGAN PARK

Glen Cove

GARVIES POINT PRESERVE

Glen Cove Creek

Mott Point

Glen Cove Avenue

Mosquito Cove

Shore Road

Prospect Avenue

Sea Cliff Avenue

Hempstead Harbor

Glen Avenue

Littleworth Lane

Downing Avenue

Beacon Hill Road

Tappen Beach Put-in

Tappen Beach

W Shore Road

Shore Road

HEMPSTEAD HARBOR PARK

Bar Beach

Glenwood Road

N

Scudders Lane

South Glenwood Landing

Mott Cove

Glenwood Road

Motts Cove Road

0   0.2   0.4   0.6 miles

0   0.2   0.4   0.6 kilometers

But while Hempstead's bordering towns enjoyed the wealth and prosperity that came with their development, the harbor began to pay the price. Its southern portion began to accumulate large amounts of silt, eventually becoming too shallow to support any large vessels. The industrial facilities in the Glen Cove area began dumping large quantities of toxic substances and waste into the creek and harbor, effectively destroying the habitat for all organisms. A power plant was opened on the harbor's eastern shore. Sand and gravel mining were carried out in earnest on its western shore. And overfishing occurred at a tremendous rate. Things got so bad that by the mid- to late 1900s, Hempstead Harbor had become one of the most polluted bodies of water on Long Island.

Thankfully, residents and local politicians realized something had to be done. They placed strict restrictions on what could be released into the water, upgraded sewage-treatment plants, fought future development plans, removed old and derelict barges, and created the Hempstead Harbor Protection Committee, which has continued to fight for and protect the harbor.

Fortunately, these steps have begun to work. Some shellfish have been restored; many bird and fish species have returned; wetland plants have rebounded; and fishermen, boaters, and swimmers have slowly but steadily come back. In recognition of its current state of rejuvenation and its overall ecological importance, New York State has even designated Hempstead Harbor as a Significant Coastal Fish and Wildlife Habitat. Citing the success of all involved in helping save the harbor, Sea Cliff Mayor Bruce Kennedy recently stated, "The results achieved through this team approach have been tremendous. There is still a lot of work to do but with this type of cooperation, the future looks good."

Many of the ongoing changes are best seen from the water. And there's no better way to get on Hempstead's water than in a kayak. You can put in at Bar Beach, Tappen Beach, and Morgan Park Beach, all of which easily put the whole of the harbor at your disposal. Hempstead Harbor may not offer the most beautiful paddling experience on Long Island, but it's come a long way and for that reason is worthy of exploration.

USGS Quadrangles   SEA CLIFF (NY)

38 **DESCRIPTION** Because Tappen Beach is about midway down Hempstead Harbor's eastern shore, you can head north or south after launching. If you've started paddling south, the first thing you'll notice is an incredibly large, formidable-looking bulkhead that protects a marina on your left. The marina's entrance is somewhat hidden from view, with an opening in the bulkhead facing south. Because of this, you may not be able to see a boat coming out of the marina until it's right on top of you, so pay attention to your surroundings as you paddle down the bulkhead's length.

The bulkhead ends in 0.5 mile, almost directly opposite Bar Beach, although the shoreline doesn't open up much after that. Instead, you'll be greeted with a few rusty boats tied to a dock and an immense power plant sitting right on the water's edge. However, if you head a bit farther, past the power plant and into the harbor's southern portion, you'll be paddling along a much prettier shore, with gorgeous houses in tree-lined yards. Unfortunately, the homes fade after 1 mile,

GPS COORDINATES

Put-in/take-out
N40° 50.230' W73° 39.183'
Tide station
Glen Cove, Hempstead Harbor, NY
N40° 51.798' W73° 39.300'

Tappen Beach to Morgan Park and Back

Level	2B
Distance	6.6 miles round-trip
Time	3 hours
Navigable months	Year-round
Hazards	Open water, boat traffic
Portages	None
Rescue access	Easy
Tidal conditions	Any
Scenery	C

leaving you in the southernmost part of the harbor among some large industrial buildings and the Roosevelt Viaduct. Head north from this point and you'll be paddling along some more industry, in the shadow of a town landfill, and beside a golf course before you reach Bar Beach and the harbor's northern section once again.

After paddling 0.7 mile along Bar Beach, you'll come to a school-bus yard and a large, unsightly sand-and-gravel-mining company on the harbor's western shore. Thankfully, these eyesores disappear as you leave the mining company behind, and the harbor's west side remains lush and green almost the entire way to Long Island Sound. As you continue in that direction, you'll likely feel a change on the harbor as it widens. The wind and wave action on the open water will become more pronounced, possibly producing some chop where there was none earlier. If that's the case, not to worry—just reverse your course.

Continuing, however, will bring you to the last point of land on Hempstead's western shore, Mott Point.

Once you're paddling off Mott Point, look to the east and you should see the white bandstand, sandy beach, and long jetty of Morgan Park. This park, 1.5 miles away, makes a great destination if you want to cross to the harbor's east side, both because it is easily visible and it has a large, welcoming beach and bathroom facilities, which may be just what you need at this point in your paddle. Just be sure to aim your bow to the right of the park's jetty and not its left: if you end up on the northern side of it, it'll take you an extra 0.25 mile of paddling just to get around it.

After Morgan Park, the next place of interest on Hempstead Harbor is the Garvies Point Preserve, immediately to the south. The preserve proper covers an area of 62 acres of woodland and meadows, but its shoreline is perhaps its most spectacular part. Its rocky beach provides a home for a wide variety of marine life, including crabs, snails, and other invertebrates as well as numerous species of algae. The beach also supports the growth of spartina grass, which acts as a hiding place for many kinds of fish. And its bluffs ooze clays—deposited here millions of years ago—in a multitude of colors.

Just south of Garvies Point, Glen Cove Creek empties into the harbor after its 1-mile run. Paddle up this creek if you wish, but be warned: it's not very scenic, with more docks, factories, and warehouses than sandy beaches and trees. I recommend skipping the creek altogether and heading farther south along the harbor's shore. In your last 1.25 miles of paddling, you'll float past small beaches and dozens of quaint waterfront homes. Soon enough, you'll be back at Tappen Beach and your take-out.

◇ **SHUTTLE DIRECTIONS** To get to your put-in at Tappen Beach, take the Long Island Expressway (I-495) to Exit 37N and pick up Mineola Avenue off the service road. Travel north on Mineola Avenue 1.2 miles until it meets NY 25A. Turn right onto NY 25A and head east 0.7 mile before turning left onto Bryant Avenue. Head north on Bryant Avenue 0.9 mile, then take the left fork onto Glenwood Road when the two roads meet. Glenwood Road will end after 0.6 mile, at which point you should turn left onto Scudders Lane. Then take your second right onto Shore Road and follow it north 1 mile, looking for the parking lot for Tappen Beach on your left.

---

39 JONES BEACH STATE PARK

◇ **OVERVIEW** Certain names hold special meaning for those who call Long Island home. "The Long Island Expressway" is one. "Fire Island" and "The Hamptons" are two more. "Jones Beach" is most certainly another. Most Long Islanders have been to Jones Beach at one time or another. And even those who haven't certainly know about it. Lining the westernmost 10 miles of Jones Island, this is the most heavily visited beach along the entire East Coast, and one of the most beautiful beaches in the world.

Surprisingly, Jones Beach wasn't created by nature. Rather, it was the brainchild of real estate developer extraordinaire Robert Moses, who first saw the potential in the low-lying marshy area in the 1920s. Moses opened the park nine years later after building up the height of the land from 2 to 12 feet above sea level, stabilizing its sand by planting beach grass, constructing numerous buildings and a 2-mile boardwalk, erecting the now-iconic water tower, and creating a network of parkways, among them the Wantagh and Meadowbrook, to bring visitors to the shore. Moses' planning paid off: an estimated six million people visit Jones Beach each year. While most come to enjoy its gorgeous beach and swim in the ocean, many others look to a stroll on the park's boardwalk or a seat at an outdoor concert for their amusement.

But Jones Beach has another, more natural side that few people make use of, much less know about. The Theodore Roosevelt Nature Center houses a small natural-history museum, maintains a nature trail, and runs numerous educational programs throughout the year. The public fishing piers afford the chance to cast a line and try for some local snapper or porgy. And there's the boat basin, where you can tie up a boat for a bit and enjoy all that the park has to offer.

It's the beach's boat basin that is of most interest to kayakers, as this is the

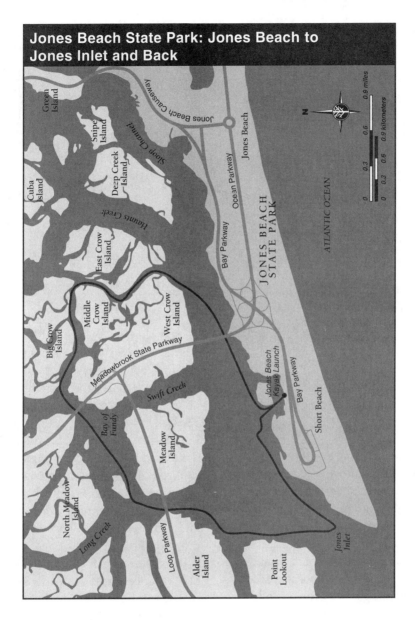

Jones Beach State Park: Jones Beach to Jones Inlet and Back

Green Island

Snipe Island

Cuba Island

Deep Creek Island

Sloop Channel

Jones Beach Causeway

Haunts Creek

East Crow Island

Middle Crow Island

Big Crow Island

West Crow Island

Meadowbrook State Parkway

Swift Creek

Bay of Fundy

Meadow Island

North Meadow Island

Long Creek

Loop Parkway

Alder Island

Point Lookout

Jones Beach Kayak Launch

Ocean Parkway

Bay Parkway

Jones Beach

JONES BEACH STATE PARK

ATLANTIC OCEAN

Bay Parkway

Short Beach

Jones Inlet

0.9 miles
0.3   0.6   0.9 kilometers
0   0.3   0.6   0
N

site of the park's kayak launch. Enter the water there, and you have instant access to the Atlantic Ocean via Jones Inlet or the vast maze of marsh islands between Jones Beach and mainland Long Island. Paddle during the late spring and summer and you'll see hundreds of common terns diving for a quick meal of baitfish, scores of herring gulls scavenging for a bite to eat, a nonstop stream of charter boats ferrying hopeful fishermen to the fishing grounds nearby, and, if you're lucky, maybe even a white pelican or two.

The boat basin is also a popular put-in for the winter paddling crowd, especially those looking to paddle among the fairly large population of harbor seals that spend the season in the waters nearby. Other wintering species include birds such as brant, common and red-breasted mergansers, and long-tailed ducks. Snowy owls have even been spied atop the dunes of Jones Beach on cold, wintry days.

Although the water around Jones Beach offers almost endless paddling possibilities, the powerboat still reigns supreme here. For this reason, you should exercise great caution whenever you kayak near the park, especially during the busiest parts of boating season. Only experienced paddlers should attempt to cross the channel when boat traffic is at its peak, and then only when conditions are just right.

USGS Quadrangles
Jones Inlet (NY)

39 DESCRIPTION Although the beach you're launching from is dedicated for kayak use, it puts you on the water along an incredibly busy part of the state boat channel, quite near the even-busier Jones Inlet. For this reason, many paddlers opt to head north immediately from the beach, scooting quickly into the widespread collection of large marsh islands across the way. This decision can be a wise one in light of the boat traffic and strong tidal currents that you may face closer to the state park. On the other hand, should you find yourself paddling here on a calm day when the channel is relatively quiet, a trip toward the inlet and possibly out onto the Atlantic Ocean may definitely be in order.

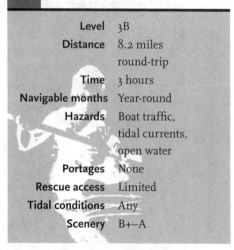

Jones Beach to Jones Inlet and Back

Level	3B
Distance	8.2 miles round-trip
Time	3 hours
Navigable months	Year-round
Hazards	Boat traffic, tidal currents, open water
Portages	None
Rescue access	Limited
Tidal conditions	Any
Scenery	B+–A

Stay close to the shore of Jones Island as you head west along the boat channel, both to stay out of the way of any powerboats and to more easily enjoy the island's natural splendor. Though only sparse vegetation grows here, the white-sand beach and abundant wildlife should be enough to capture your attention. Add the nautical charm of the commercial fishing boats that often cruise through these waters, and you'll be glad you headed in this direction first.

When you reach the inlet, take a quick glance across as the densely populated hamlet of Point Lookout comes into view. Unless you plan to paddle

GPS Coordinates

Put-in/take-out
N40° 35.399' W73° 33.114'
Tide station
Jones Inlet (Point Lookout), NY
N40° 35.202' W73° 34.698'

into the Atlantic, it's wise to cross over to the Point Lookout side of the inlet before you start your way north again. While its scenery may pale in comparison to that on the Jones Beach side, the water is quite safe here, albeit a bit shallow in some spots close to shore. In fact, a decent-sized sandbar just off the Point Lookout shore can stop your forward progress during low tides. On the upside, it can also provide you with a place for a quick rest stop.

Continue north along the beach and then cross a smaller channel as Point Lookout comes to an end. There should be only limited boat traffic coming out of this channel, so the short crossing should be uneventful. Once across, you'll be paddling along Alder Island on your way to the Loop Parkway Drawbridge, 0.5 mile distant. Once again, keep close to shore, especially as you near the bridge, to avoid any encounters with larger boats. The bridge's siren may even sound while you are fairly close to it, announcing that it will be opening for a fishing

boat or cruise ship from nearby Freeport (2 miles to the north). If that's the case, you definitely don't want to be too close when it passes you by.

You'll be turning right after you've passed under the Loop Parkway Drawbridge, sneaking between the tiny North Meadow Island and its much larger brother, Meadow Island. Look to North Meadow's western tip as you make the turn, and you'll be treated to an up-close-and-personal view of a unique South Shore structure: the iconic "bay house." While the gray home before you is just one of many such houses in existence, it's pretty indicative of their style. Most have been standing among the bay's marshes for anywhere between 30 and 100 years—amazing when you consider that they have no foundations to speak of. Instead, the homes were built on wooden platforms and were constructed out of whatever type of spare lumber could be found. Most have large porches, some sort of dock, and an eclectic assortment of

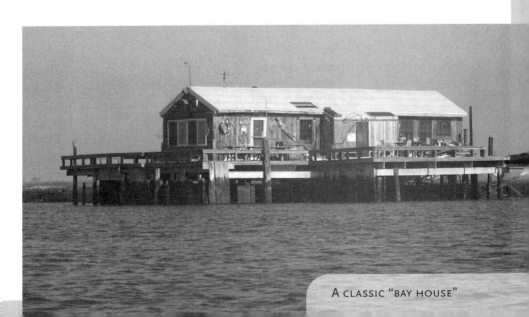

A CLASSIC "BAY HOUSE"

decorations and adornments, giving the houses charm and personality.

After passing the gray bay house, you'll be paddling in the channel that leads under the Meadowbrook Parkway Bridge and past the fairly large West Crow Island. Look to your right as you paddle past the last of Meadow Island, just before you reach the bridge, and you should see Jones Beach beyond the second Loop Parkway Bridge. If you're ready to call it a day, the 1.3-mile paddle back to the beach the option for you. Otherwise keep heading east, pass under Meadowbrook Parkway, and continue your path around West Crow Island.

You've probably noticed by this point that there is a significant amount of phragmites bordering the parkway but not much anywhere else. That's because this invasive plant is much more tolerant of poor growing conditions

and higher pollution levels than most indigenous species, and thus is better able to grow along the roadside. The majority of vegetation everywhere else consists of *Spartina alterniflora* (salt-marsh cordgrass) and *Spartina patens* (salt-meadow cordgrass). Both species can grow on or near water with a higher salt content than most other plants, hence they grow lower and more widespread than their neighbors. You might have also noticed a few isolated clusters of small trees growing near the centers of some of the larger islands you've passed—such is a sign that the land is a bit higher and drier than elsewhere, making it more suitable for some larger species.

By all means, soak up all the green scenery you can as you continue east along this stretch of water. Don't become too absorbed, though, or you may paddle past your next turn and

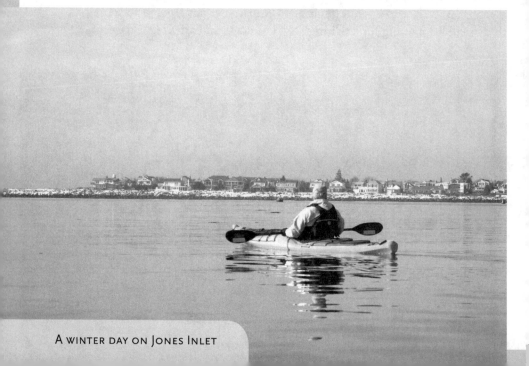

A WINTER DAY ON JONES INLET

lose your way in the confusing maze of channels. Instead, keep looking to your right (south) as you round West Crow Island and you'll notice a second, narrower channel opening up. This route will take you around the south side of Middle Crow Island and ultimately between East and West Crow. No need to worry if you miss it; you'll just have to take the next passageway south, between Middle and East Crow, which will eventually bring you to the same place.

More bay houses become noticeable in the distance as you navigate between the Crow islands. You should also see the iconic Jones Beach Tower and theatre to the south. These two structures will come in handy as guides as you find your way back to the boat basin. Once you turn southeast and seem to

be heading directly toward them, you'll have a paddle of almost 1 mile until you reach the state boat channel. Then turn right, head toward the Meadowbrook Parkway Bridge, and paddle the last 1.5 miles back to the boat basin and your take-out.

✧ **SHUTTLE DIRECTIONS** To get to the put-in in Jones Beach State Park, take the Meadowbrook State Parkway south toward Jones Beach. Pass through the toll booths, cross over the drawbridge, and look for the signs for the West End Boat Basin and the U.S. Coast Guard. Bear right and follow the signs to the boat basin. Look for its entrance after 1 mile. Once in the parking lot, follow the KAYAK LAUNCH signs to the right.

---

40   MANHASSET BAY

✧ **OVERVIEW** Considered by many powerboaters to be one of the best harbors on Long Island Sound because of its sheltered water, small tidal range, and limited current, Manhasset Bay has also taken its place among the best places on Long Island to kayak. Nestled snugly between the peninsulas of Great Neck and Cow Neck, near the border of Nassau County and the New York City borough of Queens, the bay is home to an astounding array of Gold Coast–era mansions, stately yacht clubs, waterfront restaurants, and stunning views. Consider too its narrow width (less than 2 miles) and

protected water, and you'll understand why paddlers have come to love Manhasset Bay.

Launch your boat anywhere on the bay, and you'll surely notice the stunning waterfront homes that line most of its shores and the many beautiful sailboats and yachts that sit at their docks or float on their moorings throughout its waters. While both are quite common on the bay today, things were quite different before the 1900s. In fact, the area was long used primarily as a place to catch fish and raise cattle. Such activities were so important and valuable that the European settlers changed the bay's name from the Native American *Manhansett,* or "Island Neighborhood," to Cow Bay.

With the dawn of the 20th century, the bay's focus began to change from

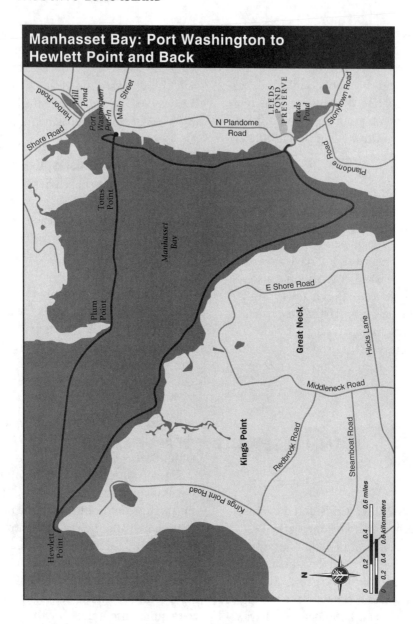

Manhasset Bay: Port Washington to Hewlett Point and Back

fish and cattle to ships and yachts. Marinas and yacht clubs appeared along its shores, more and more boats began to ply its waters, and a seaplane base opened up to service passengers coming to New York from Europe. The Long Island Rail Road also opened a station nearby, giving wealthy New Yorkers an even easier way to get out of the city and enjoy the beauty of Manhasset Bay. Eventually, the whole of the bay and its surrounding towns became synonymous with affluence—a reputation that has endured to this day.

Although you'll probably never be able to afford one of those sprawling bay-front mansions, you can easily kayak past them. The best place to begin such a trip is from the town dock in the village of Port Washington. There you'll find ample parking and easy water access, readying you to head anywhere on Manhasset Bay.

USGS Quadrangles SEA CLIFF (NY), FLUSHING (NY)

40 **DESCRIPTION** Paddling out from the town dock in Port Washington gives you three different options for exploring Manhasset Bay. Head north, and marinas, boat docks, and mooring fields will be your companions as you paddle along the Manorhaven shore. Point your bow to the west, and the Kings Point peninsula will lie before you, with the bay's mouth and Long Island Sound just beyond. Finally, paddling to the south will bring you deeper into Manhasset Bay and the attendant scenery along its shores. Though quite different, all three choices make for equally enjoyable trips. But it's the last option that is usually the most popular.

Heading south from Port Washington, you'll first encounter a series of docks sticking out into the bay. Some belong to small shipyards and others to waterfront restaurants, where boat owners can stop for a bit and get a bite to eat. Either way, this stretch of shoreline can be quite busy at times and require you to pay extra attention to your surroundings. Don't paddle too close to the ends of the docks, where you may be hidden from view, and don't cross any boat channels without checking to make sure the way is clear. Happily, this section of shoreline calms

Port Washington to Hewlett Point and Back

Level	2B
Distance	8.4 miles round-trip
Time	3 hours
Navigable months	Year-round
Hazards	Open water, boat traffic
Portages	None
Rescue access	Easy
Tidal conditions	Any
Scenery	A

down after just 0.2 mile of paddling, although a few smaller docks remain along with a large mooring field just offshore. Unfortunately, there is little room between the moored boats and the shoreline, obliging kayakers to share space with powerboaters and sailors. The area is a no-wake zone, though, so all boats' speeds should be slow enough to keep things safe.

Keep looking to your left as you paddle farther south, and the stately Port Washington Yacht Club will soon fill your view. Paddle around its docks, enjoy its many beautiful boats, and people-watch a bit you float past its grounds. Then continue south and get

GPS COORDINATES

Put-in/take-out
N40° 49.939' W73° 42.175'
Tide station
Port Washington, Manhasset Bay, NY
N40° 49.998' W73° 42.000'

ready to see one of the prettiest spots on the bay.

The 35-acre Leeds Pond Preserve is just 0.5 mile south of the Port Washington Yacht Club, at the water's edge. As you paddle up to it, you'll notice its beautiful, undeveloped shore. You'll also see the shallow, sandy delta formed by the creek that flows out of Leeds Pond. The creek is navigable during high tide, although the way onto the pond is blocked by a small dam. Nevertheless, the portion of the preserve that borders Manhasset Bay is stunning enough that you won't really miss the rest.

Past the preserve, you'll likely notice that the bay starts to narrow. If you didn't realize it already, you'll also find that the moorings have disappeared, though a few scattered docks remain. You can paddle another mile along this eastern shore before coming to the southernmost part of the bay, passing more docks and waterfront homes

along the way. This is also a good place to cross over to the western shore, as the distance is only 0.3 mile and there's little in the way of boat traffic to make it difficult.

Like its eastern counterpart, the western shore is lined with dozens of waterfront homes, although these seem to increase in size as you paddle farther north. In fact, paddling only 0.5 mile north of where you crossed the bay brings you to a stretch of shore where gorgeous mansions occupy terraced yards with elaborate landscaping. Stone fountains, sculptures, gardens, and manicured lawns seem to be the norm along this stretch of the Kings Point peninsula.

Continue paddling alongside these beautiful residences. If you can stop looking on in awe, you'll notice that the shore is beginning to curve back to the west. As it does, you will be heading almost straight toward the bay's mouth and will soon be able to see Long Island

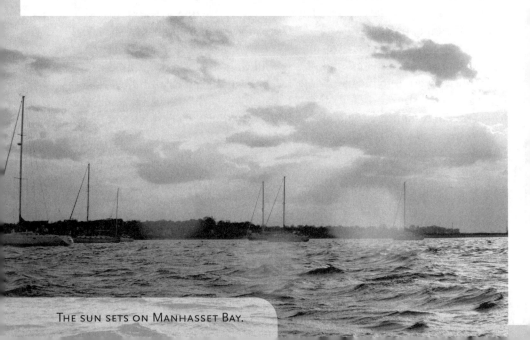

THE SUN SETS ON MANHASSET BAY.

Sound and Hart Island in the distance. From here, the last bit of land on the Kings Point peninsula, Hewlett Point, is only 2 miles distant. If you paddle this far, you'll be treated to an amazing view of the New York City skyline to the west, framed by the Throgs Neck and Whitestone bridges. You'll also have a few dozen partially submerged rocks to contend with just offshore.

With so many rocks both on shore and off, landing is almost impossible along Hewlett Point. Thankfully, there's a spot just big enough for a sea kayak or two on its western side, where a break between two rocks reveals a tiny patch of pebbly beach. Look for this spot if you need to take a quick break or stretch your legs before heading back to Port Washington. The crossing is about 3 miles long but can feel much longer since you've been sitting in a kayak for a few miles already.

Once you've soaked in enough of the view from Hewlett Point, bear toward the finger of land that you see straight ahead, Plum Point. Halfway between Hewlett Point and Port Washington, it makes a good point of reference as you cross. It can also make for a good rest stop if you need one more break before you finally make it back to the Port Washington dock.

◇ **SHUTTLE DIRECTIONS** To get to the put-in at the town dock in Port Washington, take the Long Island Expressway (I-495) to Exit 36 (Searingtown Road). Follow the exit ramp to Searingtown Road and make a right. Take Searingtown Road north 3.9 miles into the village of Port Washington. Once in the village, turn left onto Main Street and follow it 1 mile until you reach the water. Look for the signs indicating the parking lot for the town dock as the road curves sharply to the south.

 ## NORMAN J. LEVY PARK, MERRICK

◇ **OVERVIEW** Imagine launching your boat along the banks of a beautiful but long-forgotten brook that flows between a lush, verdant marsh on one side and a scenic nature preserve on the other. Now imagine that this slow-flowing run of water eventually carries you to a wide and expansive bay with stunning views in every direction. Along the way, you pass scores of herons, egrets, swallows, and ospreys but can also cast a line and try your luck

at landing a striped bass or bluefish. Such a place seems almost too good to be true. Thankfully, it isn't: I've just described Norman J. Levy Park and Preserve in Merrick.

The 52-acre park is an amazing place to visit—especially when you consider that it was nothing more than a town landfill 12 years ago. Its transformation into a park and nature preserve occurred under the auspices of the Town of Hempstead, whose engineer was awarded the 2002 Outstanding Engineering Achievement Award for the groundbreaking work. Instead of being closed down and capped, as is normally the case, this

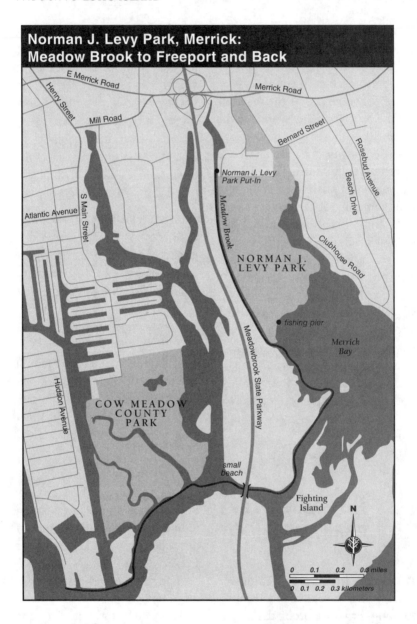

Norman J. Levy Park, Merrick:
Meadow Brook to Freeport and Back

landfill underwent a different procedure that included planting indigenous trees, shrubs, and grasses to both stabilize and rejuvenate the area. These plant species were also chosen specifically to attract wildlife to the preserve—a plan that has worked exceedingly well so far.

Near the center of the preserve stands its unique agricultural-style windmill, which generates the power needed to circulate the water in its two ponds. Three miles of hiking trails also wind throughout the preserve, an amphitheater sits ready to host any kind of presentation, and a state-of-the-art fishing pier juts out from the preserve into Merrick Bay. Even more important to paddlers, an easy-to-use kayak ramp sits right on Meadow Brook (from which the Meadowbrook Parkway got its name) just a few feet west of the parking lot. Use it to launch your own boat for free, or rent one for only $20. You can also schedule a free kayak tour of the preserve by calling 516-804-2000.

USGS Quadrangles
FREEPORT (NY), JONES INLET (NY)

41 **DESCRIPTION** As you climb into your boat and begin your trip south on Meadow Brook, you'll feel as if you've entered another world altogether. Gone is the hustle and bustle of the park with its joggers, hikers, and stroller pushers. Still water, fluttering birds, blue sky, the scent of wildflowers, and the wind rustling through the grass will be all that you experience as you make your way south toward the bay. Only about 10 feet wide for most of its run, the brook is bordered by tall phragmites on the right and a wide assortment of trees and shrubs on the hill to the left. Birch, silver and red maple, and willow trees share the area with alder bushes and the occasional tree of heaven, while pesky poison ivy fills in much of the space in between.

Continue paddling downstream, and not only will the variety of plant life astound you, but so will the multitude of birds singing, calling, and flying along the water. Great egrets, black-crowned night herons, and red-winged blackbirds will surely make an appearance; if you're lucky, ospreys, warblers, and even kingfishers may stop by as

Meadow Brook to Freeport and Back

Level	1A
Distance	5.5 miles round-trip
Time	3 hours
Navigable months	Year-round
Hazards	Boat traffic, bridges, tidal currents
Portages	None
Rescue access	Limited
Tidal conditions	3 hours before or after high tide
Scenery	A+

well. There's a bit of unfortunate road noise from nearby Meadowbrook Parkway, but even that will do little to distract you from the natural beauty of the brook you're paddling down.

After 0.5 mile of paddling, you'll be close enough to the bay that the plant life on the brook will begin to change a bit. You should notice that the phragmites that was so common upstream has started to be replaced by spartina grass and other more salt-tolerant species. The parkway will also begin to veer away from the brook, thankfully taking its noise with it. You'll see more of the surrounding area as the land

GPS COORDINATES

Put-in/take-out
N40o 38.970' W73o 33.882'
Tide station
Freeport Creek, NY
N40° 38.502' W73° 34.200'

along the water flattens out, and soon you'll have a great view of the Jones Beach Theatre and water tower in the distance. Then, after 0.8 mile of paddling, you'll finally leave the confines of Meadow Brook to float among the numerous salt-marsh islands that dominate this portion of the East Bay.

As you paddle out of the brook, stay close to the western bank and in just 0.3 mile you'll come to a channel that leads between two large marsh islands. Follow it to the southwest, and you'll soon be heading straight for the small bridge that is your gateway to Middle Bay and the canals of Freeport. Keep an observant eye along the way and you'll probably be able to add a few more bird species to your already extensive list. Common and least terns usually congregate in large numbers here, as do willets, sandpipers, swallows, and oystercatchers. In addition to

birds, keep an eye out for powerboats along this stretch of water, most of which is part of the marked boat channel. It can become quite busy during boating season.

Once you reach the small bridge that crosses the boat channel, you'll have to paddle through if you want to explore the western side of the parkway. Unfortunately, there's not much room for kayaks except that which is also used by powerboats. Given the sharp turns in the boat channel that lead up to the bridge and can hide incoming boats, passing underneath the bridge can be a daunting experience. Nevertheless, be patient, observant, and committed, and you should have no problem gaining access to the other side of the bay.

At this point, you may wish to stop and rest a while before you go any farther on the water. If so, immediately

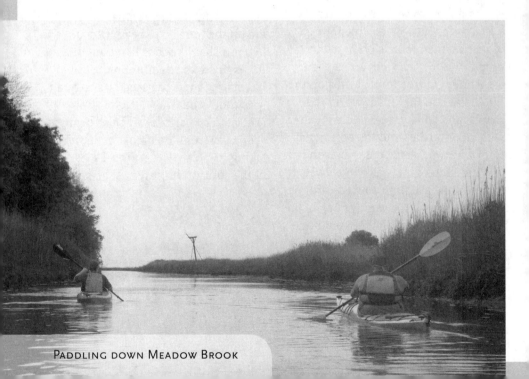

PADDLING DOWN MEADOW BROOK

to the north of the bridge you just passed under is a small, cozy beach that's good for a pit stop and perhaps a picnic. If you want to keep moving, though, the canals that make up the south shore of Freeport are excellent destinations.

The most popular canal is Freeport's "Nautical Mile," just 1.2 miles west of the bridge. Lined on its left side with scores of waterfront restaurants, bars, seafood shops, and souvenir shops, it's also home to Freeport's commercial-fishing fleet, its sightseeing cruise ships, and its gambling boats. In short, the canal is an incredibly busy stretch of water. Paddle up its length and you may find it one of the most interesting places you've ever brought your kayak. However, it can also be one of the most dangerous, on account of all the boat traffic. Keep a sharp lookout for moving boats, and be ready to stop short or turn quickly should one pull out or turn in front of you.

From Freeport's canals you can paddle farther west into Baldwin Bay or south to Jones Beach or Point Lookout. If you're not ready to leave the water just yet, you may also opt to head deeper into the maze of marsh islands south of Freeport. You could spend hours weaving and winding throughout the myriad channels among them. Otherwise, just head back the way you came, and in a little more than 2.5 miles you'll be paddling up to the kayak launch in Norman J. Levy Park.

✧ **SHUTTLE DIRECTIONS** To get to the put-in in Norman J. Levy Park, take the Southern State Parkway to Exit 22 (Meadowbrook Parkway). Get on the Meadowbrook Parkway and head south 2.8 miles before taking the M9E exit toward Merrick. Follow the exit ramp to Merrick Road and turn left. Travel 0.15 mile before turning right into the Norman J. Levy Park entrance. Once inside, follow the signs to the park and its kayak launch.

 42 **OYSTER BAY HARBOR**

✧ **OVERVIEW** "I wish that we citizens of Oyster Bay could make here a breathing place for all people of this neighborhood, especially the less fortunate ones." These words were uttered by our nation's 26th president, Teddy Roosevelt, about Oyster Bay Harbor and its shores. One of the village's most famous fans, Roosevelt loved Oyster Bay so much he moved

here in 1885 and stayed until he died in 1919. His home there, Sagamore Hill, is now a National Historic Site. Fortunately, his second wife, Edith, understood Roosevelt's love of Oyster Bay and his desire to share this love with others. The creation of what is now Theodore Roosevelt Memorial Park began at her urging.

Roosevelt would have been extremely happy to see the multitudes of people who enjoy the harbor's beauty whenever they visit this park. At the bottom of the horseshoe-shaped body of water, it boasts more amenities than Roosevelt likely would have

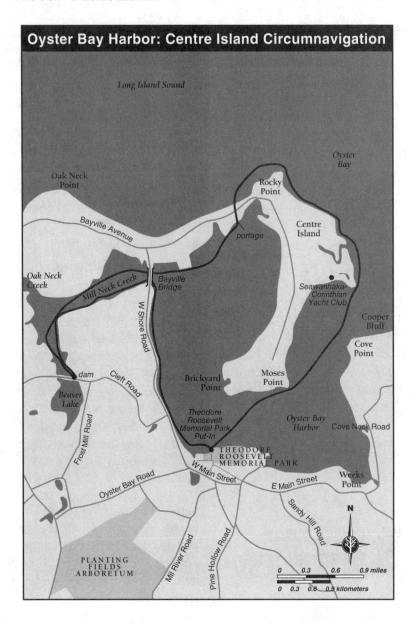

Oyster Bay Harbor: Centre Island Circumnavigation

imagined, including sports fields and tennis courts, a walking path, beach, dock, and marina, plus enough parking to support it all. An avid rower, he would also undoubtedly be pleased to know that the park has provided kayakers with a fine spot for launching their boats on the harbor's waters.

What Roosevelt and many other people both before and after him loved about Oyster Bay is completely obvious to anyone who paddles Oyster Bay Harbor. Beautiful historic buildings and sprawling waterfront homes line the shores almost everywhere one looks, while graceful sailboats ply the blue water in between. Dozens of bird species fly, wade, and swim across the harbor's breadth. Fish jump. Oysters grow. Sea turtles pass through. Seals spend the winter. Who wouldn't love a place like this?

You have many options to choose from when paddling in Oyster Bay. Its eastern and western sides are separated by a fairly large piece of land known as Centre Island (more a peninsula than an island, actually). Both provide slightly different paddling experiences, although they both make up the majority of the Oyster Bay National Wildlife Refuge.

Paddle to the west of Centre Island and you'll be on waters that are a bit more protected than those on the east. There's plenty of coastline here to keep you busy, although the small but beautiful stretch of water called Mill Neck Creek, at the harbor's northwestern corner, is more than worthy of a visit as well.

You'll find the Cove Neck Peninsula, home of Sagamore Hill, to the east of Centre Island, as well as the famous Seawanhaka Corinthian Yacht Club to the north. Cold Spring Harbor is also just a short paddle away. So whether you're looking to enjoy a bit of nature while paddling on calm and quiet waters, interested in checking out the gorgeous homes on the harbor's shores, or planning to head out of the harbor to points beyond, Oyster Bay will serve you right.

USGS Quadrangles BAYVILLE (NY)

42 **DESCRIPTION** At the harbor's southernmost end, the beach at Theodore Roosevelt Memorial Park is ideally

Centre Island Circumnavigation

Level	3C
Distance	12 miles around
Time	4–5 hours
Navigable months	Year-round
Hazards	Boat traffic
Portages	1
Rescue access	Easy
Tidal conditions	Any
Scenery	A

situated as a starting point for a paddle virtually anywhere on Oyster Bay. Kayak here during the late spring and summer, though, and most of the southern harbor will be filled with both moored and moving boats. So it's usually wise to hug the shore instead of paddling straight out onto the water. With that in mind, I usually prefer to start my trip around the harbor clockwise, pointing my bow first to the west.

As you set off with the shore on your left, you'll be heading straight for a large wooden pier that juts out from the small park at Beekman's Beach. Maneuver around its tip, taking care to avoid any boat traffic close by, and continue northwest up the left arm of the harbor. If you have a decent pair of binoculars with you, or you have

GPS COORDINATES

Put-in/take-out
N40° 52.652' W73° 32.201'
Tide station
Bayville Bridge, Oyster Bay, NY
N40° 54.198' W73° 33.000'

excellent vision, you may be able to see the Bayville Bridge from this point, it being your destination almost 2 miles distant. While it may still be beyond your sight, the road that runs parallel to the harbor's western shore will definitely not be. Called West Shore Road, it follows the shoreline closely, running its entire length to the bridge and adding an unfortunate bit of noise and distraction to an otherwise quiet and serene paddle. Adding further insult to injury is the large amount of stone riprap that has been placed along the harbor's bank in an effort to combat erosion. While it serves its purpose fairly well, it also prevents you from landing your boat on shore except wherever there is a break in the rocks.

Luckily, you'll soon reach the Bayville Bridge, which marks the entrance to the beautiful and sheltered Mill Neck Creek. Pass under the equally attractive drawbridge, beyond the two large sycamore trees that overlook the way, and you'll have left Oyster Bay Harbor and entered the waters of the creek. A couple dozen boats usually float on their moorings in this initial portion, as many others sit at the docks of the marina west of the bridge. Glance to your left and right as you paddle among these boats, and you'll likely notice that both sides are lined with homes, sitting both low on the creek's northern shore and high atop the bluff on its southern side.

The lower houses remain along the entire 1-mile stretch between the bridge and the sharp left turn that's coming up, but the houses built upon the bluff disappear after only 0.5 mile of paddling. What remains instead is a shoreline lush with green oak trees and mountain laurel shrubs. Once you make that sharp turn south, you'll notice that houses reappear, though they're much larger and their properties more sprawling than before. The half-dozen or so along this portion of the creek are simply stunning.

After paddling south on Mill Neck Creek for 0.6 mile, you'll reach a dam that holds back a beautiful body of water known as Beaver Lake. Unfortunately, there's no easy way to get your boat on the lake. Another spot on Mill Neck Creek is not only scenic but also navigable. This narrow, winding path through a marsh is part of the Mill Neck Preserve, on the outside corner of the sharp turn you made earlier. Paddle north on the creek and head northwest upon reaching the turn to find this unique but welcoming spot. Black and mallard ducks, along with geese and a circling hawk or two, will likely be there to greet you.

Once you've had your fill of Mill Neck Creek, you'll have to paddle back under the Bayville Bridge to get back on Oyster Bay Harbor. Stay close to its northern shore and a small town park comes into view immediately after the bridge, followed by a small marsh of spartina grasses 0.4 mile later. You'll have to decide your next move as you paddle along the marsh: you can go straight ahead to reach Centre Island and follow it south and back to your put-in, or you can go north to the causeway and portage over it to gain access to Long Island Sound. If you choose the former option, you'll be kayaking beneath homes that are just as spectacular as those on Mill

Neck Creek. In 2.7 miles you'll be at the beach you launched from. Carrying your boat over the causeway and paddling around the northern and eastern sides of Centre Island may be the more interesting choice, though it's about twice as long a trip.

A good portaging spot is just to the east of the large parking lot along the causeway. Land on the sandy beach there, and look for the short tunnel that leads under the road. Carry your boat through it and you'll be standing on the beach looking at Long Island Sound, ready to round Centre Island to the north. Do keep in mind that the sound is less protected than Oyster Bay Harbor and is thus influenced more by weather. Watch for strong gusts or large waves, and certainly do not take this route unless conditions are ideal. Otherwise, take the safer route I mentioned earlier back to your car.

If you've decided the way is safe, launch your boat and head northeast toward Centre Island's Rocky Point. The inspiration for this name should become obvious to you as you paddle along, passing some fairly large rocks that may or may not be submerged just beneath the surface. Pay attention to your surroundings and you should have no trouble navigating this stretch. After 0.7 mile, you will be rounding the point and well on your way south toward Oyster Bay.

Continue south—southeast, actually—with Centre Island to your right, and you'll come to a tiny break in the sand 1 mile later. The creek here is very paddleable during periods of high tide, corkscrewing for 2 miles almost completely across to Centre Island's western shore. You'll also encounter the famed Seawanhaka Corinthian Yacht Club, founded in 1871 and named after the Native American tribe that once inhabited Centre Island. Enjoy the gorgeous views of its clubhouse, stately yachts, and classic sailboats as you paddle past, but don't dawdle: you still have almost 2.5 miles left between you and your take-out. Luckily, most of that distance is along a stretch filled with even more luxurious homes, each seemingly bigger and more opulent than the one before.

You'll soon reach the southern tip of Centre Island, just across the harbor from the village of Oyster Bay. Point your bow southeast, look both ways before crossing the boat channel, and cross the 1-mile gap to the park and beach you launched from 12 miles ago.

✧ **SHUTTLE DIRECTIONS** To get to the put-in at Theodore Roosevelt Memorial Park, take the Long Island Expressway (I-495) to Exit 41N (NY 106/107). From the exit, take NY 106 north 6.3 miles into the village of Oyster Bay. Once in the village, turn left onto Audrey Avenue and drive 0.25 mile, following the signs to Theodore Roosevelt Memorial Park. Its entrance will be on your right, just across the train tracks. Once in the park, look for its boat ramps in the northwest corner.

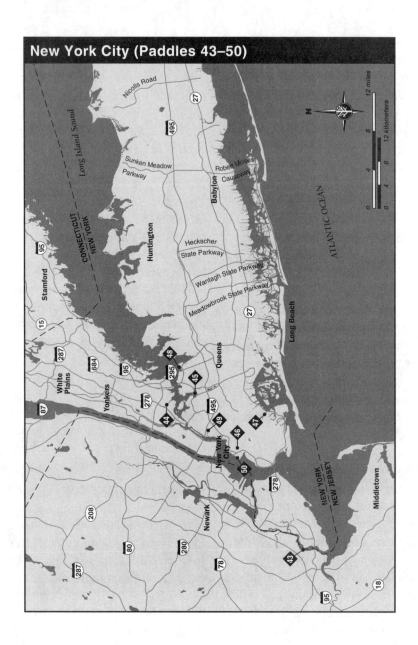

New York City (Paddles 43–50)

Long Island Sound

Nicolls Road

27

495

Sunken Meadow
Parkway

Robert Moses
Causeway

Babylon

Huntington

Heckscher
State Parkway

Wantagh State Parkway

Meadowbrook State Parkway

27

Long Beach

ATLANTIC OCEAN

CONNECTICUT
NEW YORK

Stamford

95

15

287

684

95

White
Plains

Yonkers

278

295

48

45

495

49

47

Queens

87

44

46

New York
City

50

278

NEW YORK
NEW JERSEY

Middletown

208

Newark

80

280

78

43

18

287

95

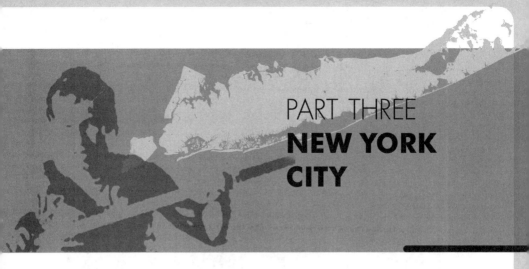

43 ARTHUR KILL

✧ **OVERVIEW** The Arthur Kill is a tidal strait on the western side of Staten Island, running between it and the state of New Jersey. It effectively cuts off Staten Island from the mainland and connects New Jersey's Raritan Bay and Newark Bay. The strait's English name is derived from the Dutch *Achter Kill,* or "Back Channel"—an appropriate designation, since the strait bypasses New York Upper Bay altogether.

Because of the shortcut it provides between New Jersey's two largest industrial harbors, the Arthur Kill has become one of the most heavily traveled bodies of water in New York Harbor. On any given day it can see dozens of tugs, barges, tankers, freighters, and container ships cruising up and down its length to Port Newark, the Atlantic Ocean, and the many oil and shipping facilities that line its banks. The Arthur Kill is also

the main thoroughfare to the now-closed Fresh Kills Landfill. Considering the nature of the waterway and the heavy industry along its length, you can see why some refer to this region of New Jersey as the "Chemical Coast."

If the Arthur Kill is so heavily traveled and the region it flows through is packed with commercial docks, oil tanks, containers, and cranes, what attractions are there for sea kayakers to enjoy? Truth be told, there are few, if any, on the strait's New Jersey side. On the other hand, the Staten Island side of the Arthur Kill is lined with salt marsh for a good portion of its length. Though small, the marshes provide a scenic place to paddle and sufficient distraction from the industry on the opposite shore. There's also the legendary Staten Island ship graveyard, which is always a draw for anyone kayaking near Rossville.

Since the 1930s, the Witte Marine Equipment Company of Staten Island has been collecting derelict ships and dismantling them for scrap and parts. Because the company's founder, John J. Witte, refused to cut up or get rid

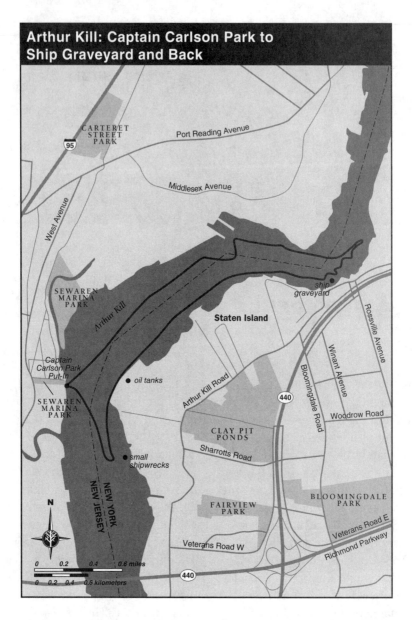

Arthur Kill: Captain Carlson Park to Ship Graveyard and Back

of any boats unless there was a buyer for them, the scrap yard eventually accumulated about 400 rotting hulks of ships, most of which were left on the muddy bottom of the Arthur Kill. When Mr. Witte passed away, the company's new management began to remove some of the wrecks, ultimately getting rid of almost 200 rotten hulls. But roughly 200 or so remain for intrepid kayakers to explore.

Truth be told, few people have ever heard of the ship graveyard, and even fewer have seen it. On the Arthur Kill, just south of the Fresh Kills Landfill, it isn't visible from any roads or other public places. The only way to see it, in fact, is from the water. If you want to experience it for yourself, you can launch from a New York City Water Trail site on the Arthur Kill. The launch is at the southern tip of Staten Island in Conference House Park, about 5.5 miles from the graveyard, though some people may find this put-in a bit too distant. Happily, a second, more popular put-in lies on the New Jersey side of the Arthur Kill in Sewaren. Indeed, most visitors to the ship graveyard begin their paddle here, at Captain Carlson Park. Only 2 miles from the sunken ships, it has restrooms, picnic tables, and a convenient boat ramp.

Whether you start from Captain Carlson Park or Conference House Park, you should exercise great caution in paddling to and around the ship graveyard. As mentioned before, the Arthur Kill is incredibly busy, with almost continuous boat traffic cruising its length. To have a safe trip, you'll need to be very mindful of your surroundings and any other boats nearby. Likewise, once you've reached the graveyard, pay close attention to where you're paddling—rotten timbers, scraps of metal, and pieces of rope, rubber, glass, and other debris lie strewn about, ready to snag you or your boat as you float by. If you can, kayak here with others, and keep a safe distance from the wrecks.

USGS Quadrangles
PERTH AMBOY (NJ), ARTHUR KILL (NY)

43 **DESCRIPTION** As you look out on the Arthur Kill from the ramp at Captain Carlson Park, the first thing you'll probably see is the collection of large oil tanks directly across the strait

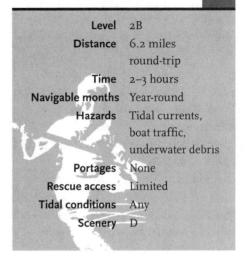

Captain Carlson Park to Ship Graveyard and Back

Level	2B
Distance	6.2 miles round-trip
Time	2–3 hours
Navigable months	Year-round
Hazards	Tidal currents, boat traffic, underwater debris
Portages	None
Rescue access	Limited
Tidal conditions	Any
Scenery	D

from you. Look to the right of them and you'll also see a large stretch of green where a small salt marsh sits at the water's edge. Follow the marsh and the lush woodland just behind it, a bit farther to the south, and something even more interesting should come into view: a small collection of ships, broken apart and left to rust and rot. Though nowhere near as extensive or exciting as the main ship graveyard farther north, this smaller version is worth an inspection and the 0.6 mile of paddling it will take to get there.

Although you can make out the outlines of the ships from the wrecks that

GPS COORDINATES
Put-in/take-out
N40o 32.709' W740 15.242'
Tide station
Rossville, NY
N40° 33.402' W74° 13.398'

sit there, determining their age and original design is a bit harder to do. The only thing that will be completely obvious is the fact that they've been sitting in the mud for quite some time. Take your time paddling around these pieces of history, and snap as many photos as you wish. But do not stay too long—there's still much more to see on the strait.

Head up the Arthur Kill's eastern shore, and in 0.3 mile you'll reach the oil tanks you viewed earlier from Captain Carlson Park. The facility that houses them occupies 0.5 mile of waterfront, after which the shore is once again mostly undeveloped. A construction yard juts out into the Kill slightly north of the oil tanks, interrupting the otherwise-unbroken shoreline. But after just a few paddle strokes, the wooded shore returns.

Once you pass the construction yard, you should notice that the shoreline begins to curve a bit to the east. Follow this curve and in a very short time you'll be heading straight for the large hills of the Fresh Kills Landfill. Paddle a bit farther and you'll see the beginning of the ship graveyard. It's hard to make out details at first—just a faint outline of what look like ships in the distance—but as you draw closer and closer, the scene before you snaps sharply into focus.

The graveyard stretches 0.5 mile along the Arthur Kill, containing the remains of about 200 ships of various designs and ages and in various states of decay. Some can easily be identified as tugboats, ferries, or tankers; others are figureless hulks of wood and metal. Some hatches are open, a few lifeboats sit in their

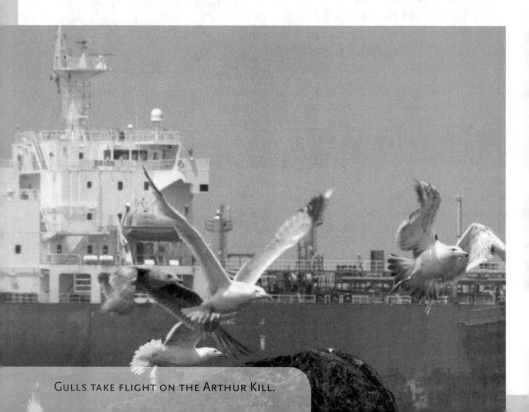

GULLS TAKE FLIGHT ON THE ARTHUR KILL.

cradles, and a couple of portholes still have glass. All in all, it's an eerie yet mesmerizing sight. The graveyard is also fraught with unseen dangers, namely parts of the ships' structures just beneath the surface. Submerged pieces of metal and wood can easily damage your boat or cause you to capsize should you unsuspectingly float over them. Again, it's wise to view the ships' ruins from a safe distance.

You'll find that time flies as you explore the haunting array of ships left to the elements. The only real concern in this is the possibility that the tide will change while you observe and take pictures, obliging you to battle it on the way back to Captain Carlson Park. So be sure to give yourself enough time to make the 3-mile trip back to your car.

◊ **SHUTTLE DIRECTIONS** To get to the put-in in Captain Carlson Park, pick up NY 440 in Staten Island and take the Outerbridge Crossing south into New Jersey. At Exit 3 (Amboy Avenue), get off and turn right onto Amboy Avenue. Head north on Amboy Avenue 0.6 mile, then turn right onto CR 654. Follow CR 654 for 0.5 mile before turning left onto State Street. Take State Street north 0.7 mile and turn right after the oil tanks onto Ferry Street. Captain Carlson Park is at the end of Ferry Street.

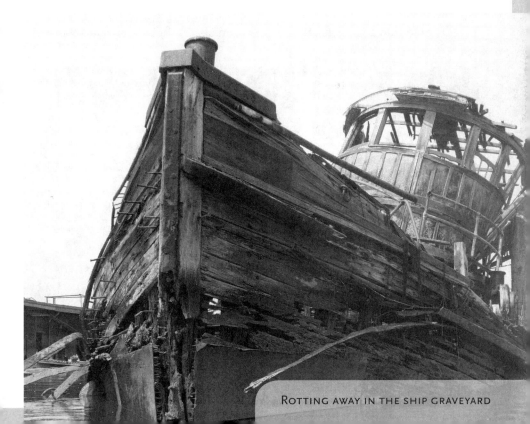

ROTTING AWAY IN THE SHIP GRAVEYARD

44 BRONX RIVER

✧ **OVERVIEW** The Bronx, New York City's only freshwater river, rises from the Kensico Reservoir, 24 miles north of the city. From there it heads south, passing through suburban and urban areas before emptying into the East River. But despite its length and prominent location, the river is often overlooked by some residents and taken for granted by others.

Since Jonas Bronck, the river's namesake, began trapping beaver there in the 1600s, the Bronx has been used and abused by humans. It's seen its share of hunting, fishing, dams, and mills. Its water has been diverted into aqueducts, its course straightened, and its banks hardened with rocks and concrete. Most detrimental, however, has been its use for carrying raw sewage. Thanks to the efforts of conservation groups like the Bronx River Alliance, though, the river has recently undergone a dramatic recovery.

The Bronx's waters are now cleaner then they've been in years. Erosion-control measures are being put into place, invasive plants such as purple loosestrife and Japanese knotweed are being removed, and native plant and animal species are returning. In fact, paddling the river is like entering another world—an oasis in the middle of a city. Beautiful red maple, red oak, and sycamore trees tower over the many ducks, turtles, and small baitfish swimming in the river. Alewives have been successfully reintroduced in the

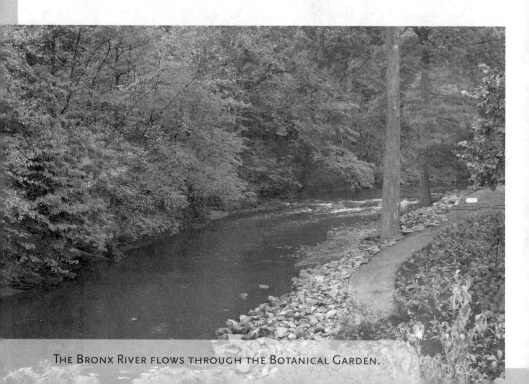

THE BRONX RIVER FLOWS THROUGH THE BOTANICAL GARDEN.

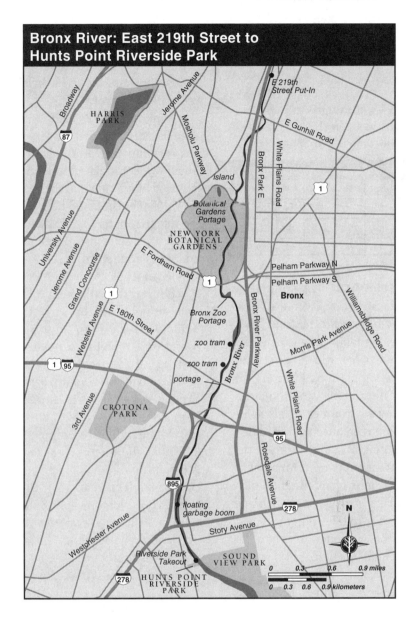

Bronx River: East 219th Street to Hunts Point Riverside Park

Broadway

87

HARRIS PARK

Jerome Avenue

Mosholu Parkway

E 219th Street Put-In

E Gunhill Road

White Plains Road

Bronx Park E

Island

Botanical Gardens Portage

NEW YORK BOTANICAL GARDENS

University Avenue

Jerome Avenue

Grand Concourse

E Fordham Road

1

Pelham Parkway N

Pelham Parkway S

Bronx

Williamsbridge Road

1

Webster Avenue

E 180th Street

Bronx Zoo Portage

Bronx River Parkway

zoo tram

Morris Park Avenue

1 95

zoo tram

portage

Bronx River

White Plains Road

3rd Avenue

CROTONA PARK

95

895

Rosedale Avenue

278

Westchester Avenue

floating garbage boom

Story Avenue

N

Riverside Park Takeout

SOUND VIEW PARK

278

HUNTS POINT RIVERSIDE PARK

0   0.3   0.6   0.9 miles

0   0.3   0.6   0.9 kilometers

river and can also be seen swimming its waters. Even a couple of beavers have made a home on the river for the first time in over 200 years.

The natural diversity of life on the river is amazing. Furthermore, the chance to paddle through the New York Botanical Garden and the Bronx Zoo makes the Bronx River a great place to paddle. The Bronx River Alliance has started running kayak tours for all who want to experience it for themselves. Visit **bronxriver.org** for more information. The New York City Parks Department has also included two kayak-launch sites on the river as part of its water trail. For a map, go to **nycgovparks.org/facilities/kayak.** In short, there's never been a better time to paddle the Bronx River.

USGS Quadrangles
MOUNT VERNON (NY),
FLUSHING, CENTRAL PARK (NY)

Mean Water Temperatures by Month (°F)						
	JAN	**FEB**	**MAR**	**APR**	**MAY**	**JUN**
MEAN	42	47	54	59	63	73
	JUL	**AUG**	**SEP**	**OCT**	**NOV**	**DEC**
MEAN	75	75	71	60	50	41

44 **DESCRIPTION** The northernmost put-in on the Bronx River is at Shoelace Park on East 219th Street. The river is very shallow at this point and only about 25 feet wide. It also runs very close to the Bronx River Parkway here, creating a noisy and somewhat distracting environment. This noise will be forgotten after a few paddle strokes, though, as the beauty of the river becomes apparent. Amazingly, almost all signs of apartment buildings and city streets are easily hidden behind silver maple and sycamore trees, some wide enough to be at least 100 years old. You'll feel as if you've left the city altogether.

The river is also incredibly straight in this section as a result of decades-old attempts at controlling its flow. Unfortunately, the modification of the route has led to considerable erosion along the river's banks, which has in turn led to the proliferation of a plant called Japanese knotweed, which the World Conservation Union has listed as one of the world's 100 worst invasive species. Look left or right along

this stretch of river and you'll surely see it: it's easily identifiable by its wide, heart-shaped leaf and small spike of whitish flowers, as well as its telltale walls of dense growth.

Thankfully, the Bronx River Alliance has spearheaded conservation and restoration efforts along the river. Small wooden stakes pounded into the mud along much of the river here slow down erosion and help maintain the integrity of the riverbanks. The group has also begun to remove the knotweed and reintroduce indigenous species in its place.

The river flows through this artificially straightened course for 0.5 mile until it makes a sharp left turn and passes under the Bronx Boulevard overpass. It then begins to twist and turn as it continues south, eventually coming to a small island 1 mile later. Both sides are navigable, although the path to the right is recommended. Not long after, the Bronx passes between two sections of green fencing on both banks. This marks the northern boundary of the New York Botanical Garden. Although it is very tempting, landing boats within the garden's property is prohibited. The Bronx is perhaps its most beautiful at this

GPS COORDINATES

Put-in
N400 43.381' W730 08.863'
Take-out
N400 49.076' W730 52.886'
Tide station
Westchester Avenue Bridge,
Bronx River, NY
N40° 49.998' W73° 52.998'

East 219th Street to Hunts Point Riverside Park

Level	1A
Distance	5.5 miles one-way
Time	3 hours
Navigable months	Year-round
Hazards	Strainers, underwater debris
Portages	3
Rescue access	Easy
Tidal conditions	Any; largely rain-dependent
Scenery	B

point, though, so most paddlers would not want to leave it anyway.

Much of the old-growth forest within the garden is visible from the river. Some of the tallest tupelo and willow trees you may have ever seen will keep you company as you paddle through the property. Don't get too wrapped up in the scenery, though—your the first portage of the trip comes 0.5 mile after you've passed between the fences. The garden's staff has created a short marked trail to help circumvent the waterfall there. The trail starts on the left riverbank, just before the signs warning of the falls. Follow it to a spot downriver where you'll reenter the water.

Once you're back on the river, a few hundred feet of paddling will bring you under another overpass, marking the southern boundary of the New York Botanical Garden and the beginning of the Bronx Zoo property. As with the garden, the zoo prohibits visitors by water. Paddlers who disregard

this rule may find themselves in trouble with zoo staff and perhaps some angry animals. However, paddling through the middle of the zoo is an experience not soon forgotten.

You'll reach a second waterfall 0.25 mile after entering the zoo property, requiring another portage. The waterfall is near the bison exhibit—the smell of the bison usually tips boaters off to the portage before the sight or sound of the falls does. The small island in the center of the river is the best place to land boats and carry them downriver of the waterfall. The river then flows through a much wider area, where aquatic plants like water willow, arrow arum, and cattails dominate the scene—and where two beavers, affectionately named Justin Beaver and José, have taken up residence. Keep an eye out for gnawed tree trunks, fallen saplings, and perhaps even Justin and José themselves. After another 0.5 mile, the river then passes under the zoo's monorail, where paddlers can wave to its passengers as they pass overhead.

The Bronx flows through more-developed areas once it leaves the zoo property. You must deal with one final waterfall before entering this new stretch of river, though. Boats can be landed on the right riverbank soon after passing under the second monorail track, where a rockslide helps lower paddlers and their boats to the base of the falls. From this point on, the river passes large buildings, flows under railroad and subway overpasses, and runs next to highways. It also provides one final surprise to paddlers accustomed to more-pristine environments: a floating garbage boom. This plastic-and-rubber barrier prevents garbage on the river from flowing farther downstream. Although there may be a fairly large backup of floating debris behind it, the boom is quite easy to paddle over. It also makes for a unique photo opportunity and some good paddling stories.

The river then continues south for an additional 0.5 mile before reaching Hunts Point Riverside Park. Boaters may choose to end their trip at this point or continue paddling south toward the East River. In doing so, they will have views of New York's LaGuardia Airport, the jail at Rikers Island, and Shea Stadium. This option adds 2 extra miles to the trip.

✧ **SHUTTLE DIRECTIONS** To get to the put-in at Shoelace Park, take the Bronx River Parkway north to Exit 9 (Gunhill Road). Head east on Gunhill Road, turning left onto Olinville Avenue after 0.1 mile. Olinville Avenue will take you to East 211th Street and a stop sign. Turn right at this stop sign onto Bronx Boulevard, and head north to East 219th Street. Shoelace Park's boat launch is on the river directly across from East 219th Street.

To get to the take-out at Hunts Point Riverside Park, take the Bronx River Parkway south to Exit 2W. Turn left onto Morrison Avenue, which will quickly lead to Bruckner Boulevard. Turn right onto Bruckner Boulevard and head west 1 mile, turning left onto Hunts Point Avenue. Hunts Point Avenue will reach Lafayette Avenue in 0.25 miles. Turn left onto Lafayette Avenue and head straight for the river. Hunts Point Riverside Park will be straight ahead.

Paddlers can also use the New York City subway system to bring them to their put-in or take-out locations. Stops very near Shoelace Park on East 219th Street and on Hunts Point Avenue can make shuttling to either end of the river easy. Subway maps and information are available at **mta.info.**

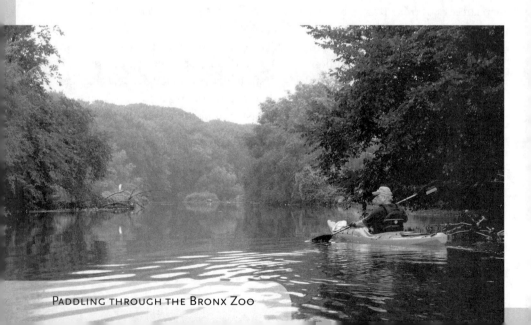

PADDLING THROUGH THE BRONX ZOO

45   EAST RIVER

⬦ **OVERVIEW** Once a polluted, unwelcoming stretch of New York City water, the East River has recently taken on new life as an immensely popular metropolitan paddling destination. Truth be told, it's not really a river at all but a tidal strait connecting the Hudson River and New York Harbor to Long Island Sound. Nevertheless, the East flows past some of New York City's prime real estate, like LaGuardia Airport, Rikers Island, Roosevelt Island, the United Nations Building, South Street Seaport, and the Brooklyn Bridge, giving all who ply its waters a lot to look at.

With the river's ever-increasing popularity among kayakers and the launching of the New York City Water Trail, gaining access to the East has never been easier. In fact, there are at least nine different launch sites associated with the water trail. Even so, paddling here is not without its dangers. Bustling boat traffic, strong tidal currents, and the infamous waters of Hell Gate can combine to make navigating the river quite an adventure. To make the most of your trip, keep the following in mind: stay out of the boat channel and you will avoid most, if not all, powerboats; follow the tidal flow to avoid paddling against the strong current; the treacherous waters of Hell Gate calm down enough during the slack between high and low tides to make paddling through them easier

and safer. The tide and current predictions listed at **tidesandcurrents.noaa.gov** show exactly when such opportune conditions occur. So whether you're participating in one of the Long Island City Community Boathouse's organized paddles or going it alone, the East River is one paddling destination not to be missed.

USGS Quadrangles
FLUSHING (NY), CENTRAL PARK (NY), BROOKLYN (NY)

Mean Water Temperatures by Month (°F)						
	JAN	FEB	MAR	APR	MAY	JUN
MEAN	34	34	37	46	59	70
	JUL	AUG	SEP	OCT	NOV	DEC
MEAN	75	76	72	61	48	37

45 **DESCRIPTION** While not especially scenic, the first few miles of a paddle down the East River are arguably unique. Indeed, you'll spend the first mile of paddling skirting the

Flushing Bay to Brooklyn Bridge Park

Level	3C
Distance	13 miles one-way
Time	4 hours
Navigable months	Year-round
Hazards	Strong currents, boat traffic
Portages	None
Rescue access	Limited
Tidal conditions	Any (be sure to hit Hell Gate at slack tide)
Scenery	A

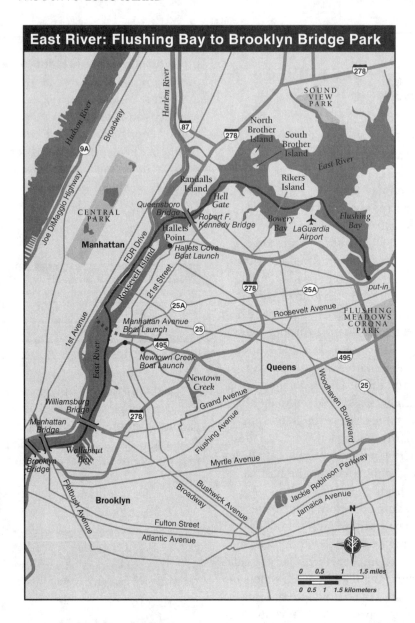

East River: Flushing Bay to Brooklyn Bridge Park

100-yard security zone of LaGuardia Airport, with passenger jets zooming overhead after taking off or on final approach for landing. Paddlers must then turn west after heading north for a mile and cruise between the airport and Rikers Island, immediately north of it. Alternately, the island can be circumnavigated. Either way, keep in mind that Rikers Island houses a very large jail (hence the barbwire fences and security cameras). Obviously, no landing of any kind is permitted anywhere on the island . . . even if you do happen to know someone who calls Rikers home.

After 4 miles, you'll have left both the airport and the jail behind while two smaller islands come into view immediately to the north (0.5 mile away). These islands, North and South Brother Island, are both uninhabited, although North Brother Island once housed a hospital where patients suffering from typhoid fever were quarantined (the infamous "Typhoid Mary" Mallon was a patient there in the early 1900s). North Brother Island is off-limits to boaters, but South Brother Island sports a small beach on its south shore that's great for a paddle break or lunch stop.

The East River continues to flow west past ten large smokestacks on the Queens shore on its way to Hell Gate, 0.5 mile later. This notorious stretch of water is known for its swift, treacherous currents and dangerous conditions that result from the confluence of three major bodies of water: the East River, the Harlem River, and Long Island Sound. As a result, only experienced and competent paddlers should attempt to navigate it, especially during its peak flow. I highly recommend paddling it only during periods of slack water. The beautiful Hell Gate Bridge comes into view soon

GPS COORDINATES

Put-in
N40° 45.627' W73° 50.968'
Take-out
N40° 42.220' W73° 59.425'
Tide station
Hell Gate, Ward Island,
East River, NY
N40° 47.202' W73° 55.302'

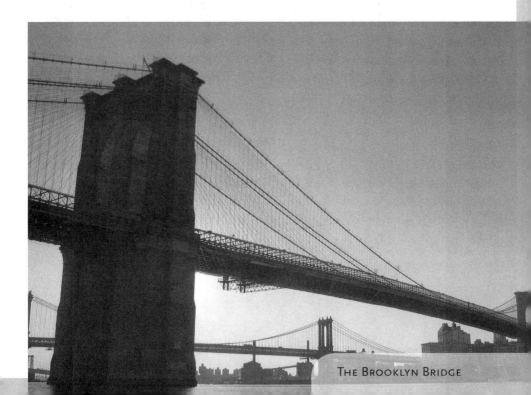

THE BROOKLYN BRIDGE

after you enter the waters of Hell Gate, with the classic Triborough Bridge spanning the East River 0.5 mile after that. Next on the river is Roosevelt Island, a 2-mile-long piece of land that splits the river down the middle.

If you want to stop and take a break or just call it a day, you can land just opposite the northern tip of Roosevelt Island, on the Queens side of the river. The Hallets Cove boat landing (part of the New York City Water Trail) is in front of the old Adirondack Furniture building. Those wishing to continue farther may head down either the east or west sides of the island, although the west side offers better views of the New York City skyline. This side also runs underneath the famous Roosevelt Island Tramway about three quarters of the way down, just north of the Queensboro Bridge.

Along with Hallets Cove, there are two more New York City Water Trail sites along the East River to aid anyone who's had enough paddling for one day. Both are on Newtown Creek, about 1 mile south of Roosevelt Island, on the Brooklyn side of the river. Beyond the creek, the East River gradually turns left and passes under the Williamsburg Bridge before it turns sharply right along Manhattan's Lower East Side. Paddlers are graced with an amazing view out into New York Harbor when heading around this right turn, with the Statue of Liberty showcased under the beautiful Manhattan and Brooklyn bridges.

The East River supplies paddlers with a surprising number of options at this point. Some may choose to continue around the southern tip of Manhattan and then up the Hudson River, while others may opt to explore the Upper Bay and possibly the Statue of Liberty. Still others may want to head farther south and take out in Louis J. Valentino, Jr. Park, in the Red Hook section of Brooklyn. Yet one more option is to land at the tiny city-park beach between the Manhattan and Brooklyn bridges. Both it and Louis J. Valentino, Jr. Park are also part of the New York City Water Trail and therefore welcome paddlers.

✧ **SHUTTLE DIRECTIONS** To get to the put-in on Flushing Bay, take the Grand Central Parkway to Exit 9E (Shea Stadium). From there follow the signs for the World's Fair Marina. The canoe and kayak launch are in the parking lot farthest to the east.

To get to the take-out in Brooklyn Bridge Park, take the Brooklyn-Queens Expressway to Exit 29 (Tillary Street). Head west on Tillary Street 0.5 mile before turning right onto Cadman Plaza West. Take Cadman Plaza West another 0.5 mile and turn right into Front Street. Head east for two blocks, then left onto Main Street. The park will be straight ahead.

46 GOWANUS CANAL

✧ **OVERVIEW** The Gowanus Canal, or Gowanus Creek Canal as it is sometimes known, is a 1.5-mile-long waterway that runs inland from New York's East River through Brooklyn's Red Hook neighborhood. Along the way, it passes numerous commercial docks, flows under five bridges, and runs alongside power plants, waste-treatment facilities, scrap-metal yards, natural-gas plants, and other forms of industry before it dead-ends at a wall of wood and concrete. Amazingly, it also provides a home to many species of birds, finfish and shellfish, aquatic plants, and the occasional mammal. Horseshoe crabs, striped bass, bluefish, herring, and jellyfish are all common sights here, and on one rare occasion a shark was spotted by numerous people. I was once even lucky enough to spot a seal playing about near the canal's mouth. That all this wildlife exists on or around water that flows through such a heavily developed area is part of the reason the Gowanus is an incredibly unique place to paddle.

Unfortunately, the canal is not without its troubles. Long used and abused by the people and businesses lining its banks, the Gowanus has accumulated more than its fair share of contaminants and pollution since it was opened in 1869. Mercury, PCBs, pesticides, and oil are just a few of the toxic substances that have been found in the canal. It is closed to shellfishing, has large amounts of litter lining its banks, and produces a stench in some spots that stems from the canal's polluted waters. The situation has become so dire that New York State recently designated the Gowanus as a Superfund site. Though it is a somewhat infamous designation, Superfund status enables the Gowanus to use state resources and funding in its cleanup and revitalization efforts.

As part of these efforts, attempts have been made to both aerate the canal's water and increase its circulation. New and improved sewer- and floodwater-discharge plans are also being developed, in hopes of restricting the amount of contaminated runoff that enters the canal. Garbage clean-ups have been held and will continue. Illegal dumping has been curbed with more enforcement. And public awareness has been raised. In fact, the Gowanus Dredgers Canoe Club has organized a walk-up paddling program which aims to get interested people out on the canal in boats. Their belief is a simple one: if people see how amazing the Gowanus Canal is, they'll be more likely to work to protect it.

While conditions on the canal are still poor, things have improved. New York City has capitalized on this improvement and has added the Gowanus to its immensely popular water trail. The canal's put-in is at the foot of Second Street, where a small wooden dock maintained by the Gowanus Dredgers sits at the water's edge, just waiting for kayakers. Paddle just one trip here, and you'll undoubtedly want to help save the Gowanus too.

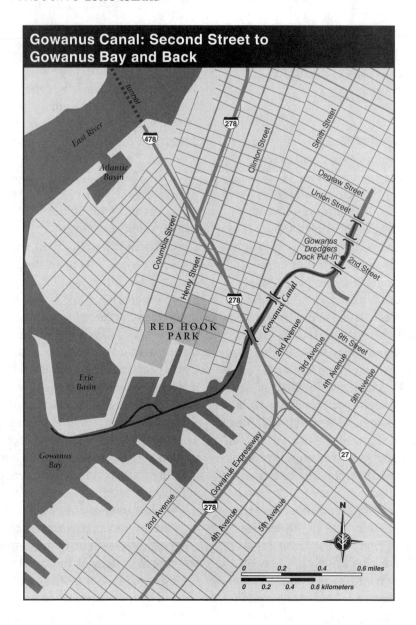

Gowanus Canal: Second Street to Gowanus Bay and Back

USGS Quadrangles Brooklyn (NY), Jersey City (NJ)

46 **DESCRIPTION** Few would call the Gowanus Canal a pretty place to paddle, but they would surely call it interesting, to say the least. This fact should become obvious to you as you launch from the Gowanus Dredgers' dock and begin heading north on its waters.

The small patch of trees directly opposite the put-in unfortunately disappears after a few quick paddle strokes, leaving you in an urban canyon of sorts, with nothing but old wooden bulkheads, warehouses, and parking lots to keep you company. You'll soon come to your first bridge just a few hundred feet to the north, with a small but unique collection of old wooden boats tied up on the left (west) side of the canal just after that. Slow down your paddling a bit and take in the unusual scenes painted on these boats—they're really something to behold. A second bridge crosses the canal just a few dozen feet north of the boats, with a fairly large floating boom blocking the way just north of that. Unless you want to tempt fate by trying to paddle over this boom and the debris it has collected, turn around and head south to see what else the Gowanus has in store.

As you retrace your paddle strokes south, you'll likely notice the series of floating white buoys and the air bubbles that seem to be rising to the surface between them. Both are evidence of a temporary system that aerates (adds oxygen to) the water, improving its health and that of the organisms living in it. Whether these efforts are working or not remains to be seen, but it's a step in the right direction regardless.

Another sign that nature is coming back to the Gowanus is the beautiful stand of birch trees on the canal's west bank, just north of the put-in. Like an oasis, these trees are a welcome sight amid the concrete and metal of the canal's neighborhood. Also encouraging are the bat boxes and birdhouses that can frequently be seen along the sides of the canal. Both seem quite successful in attracting their respective tenants.

Continue paddling past your put-in, and you'll pass under another bridge

Second Street to Gowanus Bay and Back

Level	2A
Distance	4.3 miles round-trip
Time	2 hours
Navigable months	Year-round
Hazards	Boat traffic, bridges
Portages	None
Rescue access	Limited
Tidal conditions	Any
Scenery	D

before you come to a T in the canal. Head left and you'll only be able to continue a bit before you reach a dead-end. Conversely, heading right here will eventually bring you to Gowanus Bay and New York Harbor; first, though, you'll have to paddle under a subway overpass and the Gowanus Expressway, then past more parking lots, industrial warehouses, a metal scrapyard, and a handful of barges.

The Gowanus Expressway bridge marks the end (or beginning) of what is officially the Gowanus Canal. As you paddle under it, you'll likely notice that the water feels more open now, its banks spreading apart more and more as you continue south. If the weather is clear, you should also

GPS COORDINATES

Put-in/take-out
N40° 40.615' W73° 59.389'
Tide station
Gowanus Bay, NY
N40° 39.900' W74° 00.798'

see the water of New York Upper Bay just outside Gowanus Bay, with the Verrazano-Narrows Bridge in the distance a few miles beyond. If conditions are rough, with winds stronger than you'd like, this would be an opportune time to turn around and head back to the Gowanus Dredgers dock just under 1 mile away. But if the water is calm and you're up for paddling on more-open water, continue to follow the bay's shoreline as it curves to the west, and you'll quickly be floating just off the concrete fishing pier alongside the southern border of the Erie Boat Basin.

You may be ready to pack it in at this point, in which case you'll just have to paddle the 2 miles to your put-in. If, however, you're looking for even more water to paddle, once you've passed the fishing pier you can head straight for the Statue of Liberty, just 2 miles distant, or skirt along the Brooklyn waterfront as it curves northeast toward Manhattan. You may also choose to follow the opposite side of Gowanus Bay and paddle south along Brooklyn's shore as it curves toward the Verrazano-Narrows Bridge, 4 miles away. You can't go wrong with any of these options.

⬦ **SHUTTLE DIRECTIONS** To get to the put-in at the Gowanus Dredgers dock, take the Brooklyn-Queens Expressway (I-278) to Exit 26 (Hamilton Avenue). Take Hamilton Avenue south 0.2 mile, then turn left onto Luquer Street. Follow Luquer Street 0.3 mile and it will end at Smith Street. Turn left here and take Smith Street 0.2 mile before turning right onto Second Street. Follow Second Street to the Gowanus Canal, and look for the Dredgers dock at the end of the road.

47 JAMAICA BAY

⬦ **OVERVIEW** If there's one place in the New York City area that could be considered a kayaker's paradise, it would be Jamaica Bay. Unlike most of the other locations on the New York City Water Trail, which retain their urban character despite their attempts at "getting away from it all," Jamaica Bay really does deliver when you experience it from a kayak. Wide expanses of water, vast salt marshes, numerous uninhabited islands, and a world-famous wildlife refuge are just a few of the attractions it has to offer. Consider too its great accessibility, its popularity as a prime fishing spot, and its wide variety of possible paddling trips, and its popularity among the paddling crowd is easy to figure out. Jamaica Bay is a truly amazing place, made all the more so because of its close proximity to Manhattan.

Being so close to the city has brought considerable development to the bay over the decades, namely John F. Kennedy International Airport on its east side, Floyd Bennett Field to the west, and the densely populated Rockaway Peninsula to the south. In

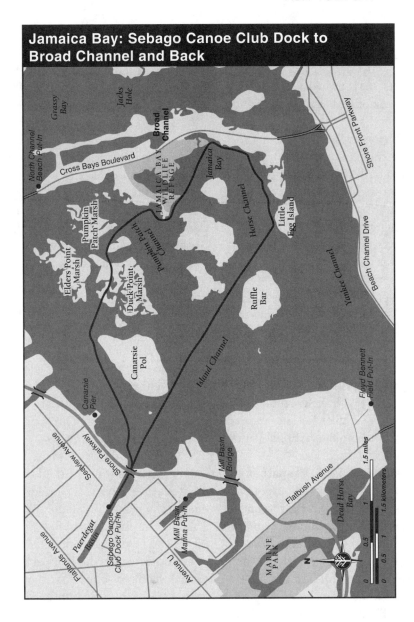

Jamaica Bay: Sebago Canoe Club Dock to Broad Channel and Back

addition, a large portion of marsh in the center of the bay was filled in and turned into the waterfront neighborhood of Broad Channel in Queens. Still, much of Jamaica Bay remains as it was when the Lenape Indians first settled along its banks hundreds of years ago.

It was this Native American tribe, not the Caribbean island, that gave the bay its name (*Jamaica* is a corruption of the Lenape word for "beaver," *jameco*). It was also this tribe that first recognized the bay's incredible productivity. As an estuary containing waters of varying salinities, Jamaica Bay sustains a wide array of organisms, ranging from striped bass and bluefish to aquatic invertebrates, crustaceans, and shellfish. It provides a home to a large group of seals each winter and a place for diamondback terrapins to lay their eggs every summer. It also acts as a stopping point for migrating monarch butterflies and supports the growth of such shore plants as beach plum, autumn olive, little bluestem, and switchgrass.

But it is Jamaica Bay's bird population that is truly remarkable. Because the bay's salt marshes make the perfect resting spot for migrating birds, an incredible number of individuals from more than 325 different species stop here at some point throughout the year. Thankfully, a large portion of this ecologically significant area was protected in 1953 with the creation of the Jamaica Bay Wildlife Refuge, and was incorporated into the National Park System in 1973.

Because Jamaica Bay is part of the New York City Water Trail, experiencing its splendor for yourself has never been easier. You can choose from four different launches, sitting in their respective corners of the bay. To the northwest is the Mill Basin Marina put-in, and to the northeast is North Channel Beach. To the south lie Floyd Bennett Field, on the bay's western shore, and the Bayswater put-in, on its eastern one. Any of these sites will serve you well as a starting point for a trip around the bay. The Sebago Canoe Club, which makes its home on the Paerdegat Basin in the bay's northwestern corner, may also be available for a paddle should you be so inclined.

USGS Quadrangles
BROOKLYN (NY), CONEY ISLAND (NY), JAMAICA (NY), FAR ROCKAWAY (NY)

47 **DESCRIPTION** As you leave the Sebago Canoe Club dock on the Paerdegat Basin, you may have trouble imagining that a wildlife refuge sits only a short paddle away. The neighborhood leading up to the club is decidedly urban: the basin is lined with marinas, and there's quite a bit of boat traffic coming and going on its waters. Head just 0.5 mile to the southeast, though, and passing under the Belt Parkway Bridge will seem like passing through a gateway to another world. Once beyond its span, you will have a great view of Jamaica Bay and will learn just how vast and expansive the bay really is. You may even see some of the dozens of bird species that make the area a world-renowned birding spot. In short, you'll be very happy you came here.

As you paddle out into the bay, glance over your right shoulder and you may see a horseback rider or two along the beach. If you do, they're likely from the Jamaica Bay Riding Academy, which offers its riders 400 acres of land and 3 miles of beach. Look to your left and you'll also be able to make out Canarsie Pier, a spot popular among the fishing crowd. The pier is also home to another New York City Water Trail put-in on the bay. Paddle between it and Canarsie Pol, the large island to your right, and you'll be ready to turn east toward the center of the bay in just 1 mile. If you can avoid hugging the beach on Canarsie Pol along this stretch, please do so—at its northernmost tip is a low nest that contains a breeding pair of ospreys.

Round Canarsie Pol and pass the osprey nest, and you'll be heading straight for some smaller areas of marsh grass that can barely be described as islands. Labeled Elders Point Marsh, Duck Point Marsh, and Pumpkin Patch Marsh on local charts, all are a sign of an unfortunate problem occurring within the bay. For reasons that scientists can only speculate about, Jamaica Bay is losing about 40 acres of marshland each year. Some blame it on the negative effects of dredging, while others believe it has to do with excess amounts of nitrogen in the water. Whatever the true reason is, these three marshes, along with many others in the area, are shrinking at an alarming rate. Thankfully, local, state, and federal governments are looking into the problem. One potential solution, begun in 2010, is to replant the area with marsh grasses and other native plants to stabilize the soil and help other species take root. Should you paddle here and encounter a large orange fence surrounding a section of marsh, you can be sure it has to do with this restoration project.

Despite losing area, these marshes contain an impressive collection of bird species, including brants, buffleheads, common terns, and many oystercatchers. Egrets are also common here, as are laughing and herring gulls and great black-backed gulls. Yet this variety of species pales in comparison to the number at the Jamaica Bay Wildlife Refuge, just 1 mile to the southeast.

If you have time, land your kayak on the beach of the wildlife refuge and take a walk around its West Pond. You'll be greeted with a well-groomed trail, informational signs, park benches, and an incredible number of bird species that are amazingly easy to observe. Everything from ibises to warblers and egrets to owls can be seen here. The area is also an important site for breeding diamondback terrapin turtles. Explore just a bit of the trail here and you'll surely want to see more. If so, go to the refuge's visitor center, where you can find informative displays, maps, pamphlets, and books. There are also bathrooms and a wildlife-viewing area.

Sebago Canoe Club Dock to Broad Channel and Back

Level	3C
Distance	11.1 miles round-trip
Time	4 hours
Navigable months	Year-round
Hazards	Open water, boat traffic
Portages	None
Rescue access	Limited
Tidal conditions	4 hours before or after high tide
Scenery	B+

GPS COORDINATES

Put-in/take-out
N40° 37.579' W73° 54.277'
Tide station
Canarsie, Brooklyn, NY
N40° 37.800' W73° 53.100'

If you can bring yourself to leave this wonderful refuge, another of Jamaica Bay's unique locations lies waiting just 1 mile farther south: the community of Broad Channel. On the southern end of the island called Rulers Bar Hassock, this charming community of bungalow-style houses sits atop a massive amount of fill and contains no less than nine canals leading inland. Each of these canals is navigable by kayak, and many of their inhabitants are often more than happy to share a hamburger or piece of chicken from their cookout as you paddle past. Some may even let you land your boat on their dock so you can stroll around town—be sure to ask first, though.

Broad Channel stretches south for 0.5 mile, leading to the southern portion of Jamaica Bay near the Rockaways. More marshes exist in this stretch of bay, as do a handful of small islands high enough to allow landing. Little Egg and Ruffle Bar are two that make great spots to stop and stretch your legs or have a picnic lunch before heading back to the Paerdegat Basin. Considering that the return trip involves a 4-mile crossing from this point of the bay, a quick break and a bite to eat may be a good idea.

On the trip back you'll be paddling through the center of Jamaica Bay, heading northwest toward your starting point at the Sebago dock. While you won't be able to see the Paerdegat Basin from Little Egg or Ruffle Bar, you should be able to make out the New York City and Jersey City skylines in the distance. Simply head northeast toward a point between them, and soon you'll be close enough to make out the Belt Parkway Bridge and the entrance to the basin. Then just paddle the last 0.5 mile

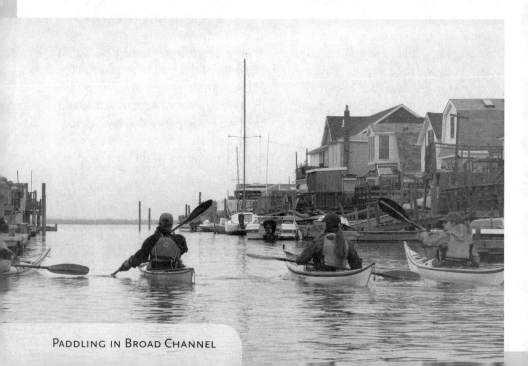

PADDLING IN BROAD CHANNEL

back to the dock, climb out of your boat, and revel in the experience you just had on Jamaica Bay.

✧ **SHUTTLE DIRECTIONS** To get to the put-in at the Sebago Canoe Club dock on the Paerdegat Basin, take the Belt Parkway to Exit 13 (Rockaway Parkway). Follow Rockaway Parkway northwest 0.5 mile and turn left onto Avenue M. Stay on Avenue M 0.9 mile until it meets Paerdegat Avenue North. Turn left onto Paerdegat Avenue North and take it 0.15 mile, at which point you should see the gates for the Sebago Canoe Club on your right.

48 LITTLE NECK BAY

✧ **OVERVIEW** Little Neck Bay is a relatively small body of water that sits in a fairly significant location. On Long Island's North Shore, about 8.5 miles east of Manhattan between Willets Point and Kings Point, it makes up part of the boundary between Queens and Nassau County. It also marks the westernmost end of Long Island Sound and the beginning of the East River, making it a strategically important body of water. In fact, part of the reason that the European settlers constructed Fort Totten on the western side of Little Neck Bay was to protect the bay and its neighboring waters from attack.

Thankfully, the defense of the bay was never challenged. It has preserved a place for itself in history, though, albeit for a different reason: as the inspiration for the name given to tiny hard-shell clams. These bivalves were harvested in great numbers from the bay during the mid- to late 1800s and became famous throughout New York and parts of Europe for their delicious flavor. Eventually, these smaller clams were called "littlenecks," after the bay in which they were originally found. Although the bay is now closed to commercial shellfishing due to pollution, many of these tiny clams are still gathered and transplanted to other areas to help rejuvenate the population elsewhere.

In addition to being a haven for littleneck clams, Little Neck Bay is also quite important to striped bass, which come to its shallow, estuarine waters in large numbers to feed and breed. Kayak here anytime between April and October, and you'll likely see a fin flip or tail splash as the bass come to the surface to catch their prey, baitfish. You'll also encounter dozens of fishermen on shore, in powerboats, and in kayaks trying to land one of these hungry predators. Paddle here in the winter and you'll be greeted by completely different wildlife and waterfowl. Scaup, mergansers, canvasbacks, and common goldeneye ducks all frequent the bay's waters when the weather turns too cold farther north.

Because it's small and protected, Little Neck Bay is a great place to paddle. Two put-ins, both part of the New York City Water Trail, sit on the

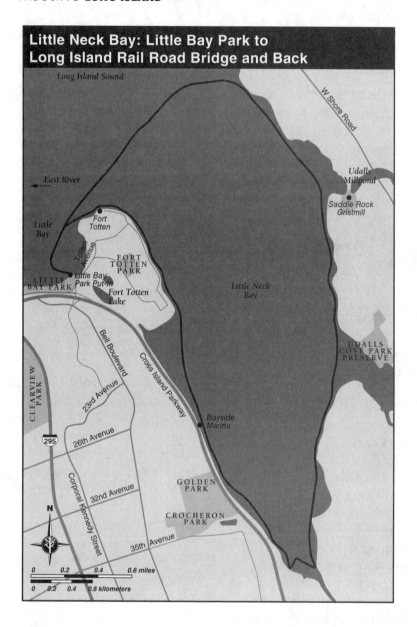

Little Neck Bay: Little Bay Park to Long Island Rail Road Bridge and Back

Long Island Sound

W Shore Road

East River

Udalls Millpond

Saddle Rock Gristmill

Little Bay

Fort Totten

FORT TOTTEN PARK

Little Neck Bay

LITTLE BAY PARK · Little Bay Park Put-In

Totten Avenue

Fort Totten Lake

Bell Boulevard

Cross Island Parkway

UDALLS COVE PARK PRESERVE

CLEARVIEW PARK

23rd Avenue

295

26th Avenue

Corporal Kennedy Street

32nd Avenue

N

Bayside Marina

GOLDEN PARK

CROCHERON PARK

35th Avenue

| 0 | 0.2 | 0.4 | 0.6 miles |
| 0 | 0.2 | 0.4 | 0.6 kilometers |

western shore, just off the Cross Island parkway. The first is at the Bayside Marina, the second near the Fort Totten entrance in Little Bay Park. Before you launch, don't forget to check the tide tables—Little Neck Bay is quite shallow and becomes a vast mudflat in some sections during low tide.

USGS Quadrangles FLUSHING (NY)

48 DESCRIPTION Launch your boat from the beach at Little Bay Park and head around the breakwater that juts out into Little Bay. You'll have an amazing view of the Throgs Neck Bridge as it crosses from Queens to the Bronx less than 1 mile away. Paddle out to the bridge, and you'll actually be on the East River instead of Long Island Sound. From here you can continue to Throgs Point and the campus of SUNY Maritime College or head down the East River, pass under the Whitestone Bridge, and paddle toward Flushing Marina near LaGuardia Airport and Rikers Island prison. But if you're looking to kayak on Little Neck Bay, turn your bow northeast and head around Willets Point, to your right.

As you round this peninsula, you can't miss the gun battery that is part of the Civil War–era fort known as Fort Totten. Built on the water's edge, this formidable brick structure keeps a proud watch over the entrance to Long Island Sound and Little Neck Bay, with dozens of ports open and ready to accept the muzzle of a cannon. It's easy to imagine the fort armed to the teeth as you paddle in its shadow. It must have been an impressive sight indeed.

Past Fort Totten, paddle northeast and cross the 1-mile-wide gap that makes up the mouth of Little Neck Bay. On the other side lies the Kings Point peninsula, home to the United States Merchant Marine Academy. The USMMA was established in 1942, on what was once the estate of Chrysler Corporation's founder, Walter Chrysler, with the mission of producing officers for the Merchant Marine service and the military. The academy's cadets learn the art of navigation, seamanship, engineering, maritime law, and other disciplines essential to running a large merchant vessel. As you near the campus on your way across Little Neck Bay, you'll likely see many of the

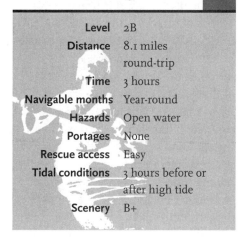

Little Bay Park to Long Island Rail Road Bridge and Back

Level	2B
Distance	8.1 miles round-trip
Time	3 hours
Navigable months	Year-round
Hazards	Open water
Portages	None
Rescue access	Easy
Tidal conditions	3 hours before or after high tide
Scenery	B+

academy's sailboats on the water or some of its larger and more impressive vessels tied to the dock. Don't paddle too close to the campus, though, as a security zone is set up around it.

To the south of the USMMA stand stately waterfront homes with sprawling lawns, elaborate landscaping, and a few docks sticking out into the bay itself. Enjoy the view of these lovely estates, then continue paddling south. Just over 1 mile south of the USMMA is Udalls Millpond, a small pond held back by the earthen dam that is part of the Saddle Rock Gristmill. This tidal gristmill, built during the late 17th century, ground grain for 240 years before it was turned into a museum. You can

GPS COORDINATES

Put-in/take-out
N40° 47.478′ W73° 46.962′
Tide station
Willets Point, NY
N40° 47.598′ W73° 46.902′

paddle right up to the mill when the tide is high enough, though the way onto Udalls Millpond is unnavigable.

The shoreline is unbroken south of Udalls Millpond, save for the small handful of private docks that jut out into the bay. Unfortunately, most of the houses that line this stretch have constructed wooden, metal, or concrete bulkheads that make landing impossible. Continue south for the next mile until you reach a small indentation in the shoreline, known as Udalls Cove. This is little more than a shallow tidal marsh, though it is the home of the Udalls Cove Park Preserve. Paddle among its grasses and you can expect to see ospreys, clapper rails, egrets, and wood ducks.

You'll be happy to see that the bulkheads that prevented landing north of Udalls Cove have disappeared south of it. Instead, this stretch of shoreline has a small but noticeable beach where you

can stop, stretch your legs, and perhaps have a bite to eat before continuing. There is also a decent-sized mooring field sitting just offshore, though plenty of room is left between it and the beach to allow a kayak safe passage.

If you're still hugging the shore at this point, you'll find that the houses disappear 1 mile south of Udalls Cove, leaving a fairly wide salt marsh in their place. This marsh has numerous channels and small creeks running through it that allow great amounts of nutrients to flow into the bay. As a result, large schools of baitfish gather in the area, which in turn attract larger predatory fish like striped bass. Paddle here anytime between spring and fall, and you'll likely run into dozens of fishermen hoping to catch one of these large bass for themselves.

You can head upstream on the largest of these creeks, which leads almost all the way to the Long Island

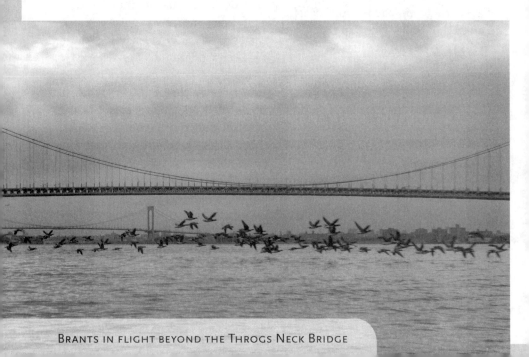

BRANTS IN FLIGHT BEYOND THE THROGS NECK BRIDGE

Expressway, or perhaps explore the maze of smaller channels that wind throughout the marsh. Heading north along Little Neck Bay's western shore is another great option. Though it is bordered by the Cross Island Parkway and experiences some road noise as a result, this stretch of shore is quite pretty, with a small rock base leading up to a line of spartina grass. In some spots phragmites grows just above the spartina, while trees block the parkway from view almost continuously.

There's little else to see along this 1.5-mile shoreline except for the Bayside Marina, 1 mile north of the bay's southern marsh. The marina has bathrooms, a snack bar, and parking that is available to everyone. It also boasts another launch site designated as part of the New York City Water Trail—this is an ideal spot for starting a paddle on Little Neck Bay if you're short on time or you want a low-mileage outing.

Once you've passed the marina, only 0.5 mile of paddling remains between you and Willets Point. Round it, and you'll have one more chance to imbibe the history of Fort Totten, soak in the beauty of the Throgs Neck and Whitestone bridges, and enjoy your view of the beginning of the East River before rounding the breakwater and paddling back to your put-in at the beach.

✧ **SHUTTLE DIRECTIONS** To get to the put-in in Little Bay Park, take the Cross Island Parkway to Exit 32 (Bell Boulevard). Get off at Exit 32 and follow the signs toward Fort Totten. Look for the Little Bay Park parking lot on the left side of the road, just before Fort Totten's entrance. The kayak launch is near the lot's northwestern corner.

49 NEWTOWN CREEK

✧ **OVERVIEW** Newtown Creek is a 3.5-mile-long side branch of the East River that runs along the border between Brooklyn and Queens. Originally a tidal estuary with a wide, slow flow, a few small islands, and a maze of channels throughout, the creek once drained many of the developing towns nearby. In fact, it got its name from one of these towns, the Dutch *Nieuwe Stad,* or "New Town." Locals fished its waters, gathered its clams and oysters, hunted its waterfowl, and used it as a means of transportation. In short, they appreciated it and all that it supplied them.

As time passed and the area became more developed, so did the creek. It grew throughout the late 18th and early 19th centuries, eventually becoming an important shipping lane in the mid-1800s, when bulkheads, docks, and a deep-water channel were constructed. This progression continued until Newtown Creek had become one of the most heavily used bodies of water in the New York City–New Jersey area.

Unfortunately, it also became one of the most polluted. With the development of industry along its banks, raw sewage, stormwater runoff, pesticides, volatile organic compounds (VOCs), and heavy metals were all dumped into

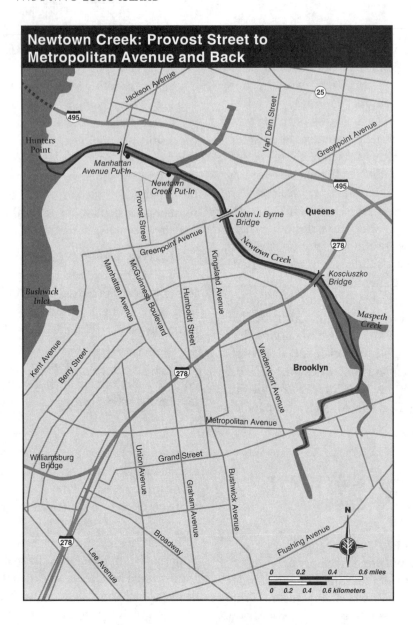

Newtown Creek: Provost Street to Metropolitan Avenue and Back

Newtown Creek at some time during its history. Sadly, few people today are even aware that an oil spill larger than the infamous *Exxon Valdez* spill in Alaska occurred on the creek in the 1970s.

Unfortunately, Newtown Creek has no natural flow other than the small tidal surge that makes its way up a small portion of its length. As a result,

it has no way to rid itself of the contaminants that build up. Instead, the creek is fed only by sewer overflow, stormwater runoff, and industrial wastewater, all of which remain mostly stagnant and add to the creek's poor conditions. Thankfully, New York State recognized the dismal situation on Newtown Creek and, in 2010, designated it as a

Superfund site, just as it did the nearby Gowanus Canal. This helps earmark state resources to help with its cleanup and restoration. Local politicians, the advocacy group called the Newtown Creek Alliance, and neighborhood residents were all overjoyed with this status, as it was a necessary step in saving their beloved creek.

Newtown Creek truly is beloved. In fact, when it was recently closed to kayaking, the local residents and paddling community created such an uproar the city had no choice but to reverse the ban and reopen the creek to paddlers. In an interview regarding the controversial closing, Assemblyman Joe Lentol made the public's views absolutely clear when he said, "I understand [the Department of Environmental Preservation's] concerns, but our constituents who use Newtown Creek understand more about the environment than they do. This really is the right thing to do. We want to encourage recreational boating in this city—it's healthy, it's green, and it encourages people to become engaged with the local waterways."

Obviously, Newtown Creek holds a special place in many people's hearts, and it should. Despite its problems, the creek is still an incredibly satisfying place to paddle. If you'd like to paddle here and enjoy its waters for yourself, you can launch from the New York City Water Trail put-in at the end of Paige Avenue in Greenpoint, Brooklyn.

USGS Quadrangles
BROOKLYN (NY)

49 **DESCRIPTION** Because the put-in in Greenpoint sits closer to the

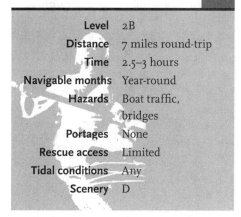

Provost Street to Metropolitan Avenue and Back

Level	2B
Distance	7 miles round-trip
Time	2.5–3 hours
Navigable months	Year-round
Hazards	Boat traffic, bridges
Portages	None
Rescue access	Limited
Tidal conditions	Any
Scenery	D

midway point of Newtown Creek than either of its ends, you must decide quickly which way to head after you launch. Look to the west, though, as you float out into the middle of the creek, and the incredible view of the Manhattan skyline will likely make that decision for you. Unfortunately, you must first paddle past a truck yard, a warehouse, a parking lot, a natural-gas refinery, and a dozen other buildings before you make it to the creek's mouth at the East River.

The scenery is decidedly urban, with little in the way of natural beauty to draw your attention. But the buildings that make up Newtown Creek's backdrop are fascinating to view from

GPS COORDINATES

Put-in/take-out
N40° 44.224' W73° 56.818'
Tide station
Hunters Point,
Newtown Creek, NY
N40° 43.998' W73° 57.000'

the water and only add to its allure. Unfortunately, such heavy development brings with it large amounts of garbage and pollution, much of which has ended up in the creek. As a result, you must swerve, dodge, and often back-paddle to avoid the sometimes large mats of floating debris that lie in your way.

The last I time I paddled here, I tried to keep a mental list of the types of trash I encountered floating along the creek. Amazingly, this list grew too long to keep track of, proving a sad reminder of how bad conditions on the creek have become. Happily, I was also able to keep another list on this same trip: a list of the bird species I observed, including Canada geese, cormorants, common terns, brants, common mergansers, a kingfisher, and a great egret. Although much shorter than the list of refuse I ran into, my list of birds is an encouraging sign of improvement on Newtown Creek.

Keep an eye out for these bird species as you continue west, and the half-mile between your put-in and Newtown Creek's only other put-in, at Manhattan Avenue Park, will pass before you know it. The creek then begins a slow curve to the south, leading you straight to the East River and the island of Manhattan. Continue to the creek's mouth and you'll be floating on the East River, just south of where the Queens-Midtown Tunnel passes underneath. From here you can easily ride the incoming tide north to Roosevelt Island and the waters of Hell Gate, or you can use an outgoing tide to carry you south toward the Brooklyn Bridge and South Street Seaport. You can also just float, soak in the city views, and head back up the creek whenever you're ready.

Once you've retraced the mile of paddle strokes between the East River and your put-in, you'll notice a small arm of water branching off the creek to your north. While it may look appealing, the branch is unnavigable due to a low railroad bridge that crosses it farther upstream. Just beyond this branch

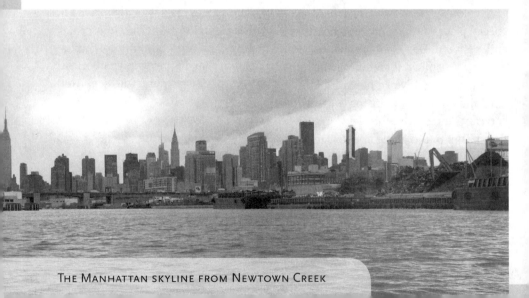

THE MANHATTAN SKYLINE FROM NEWTOWN CREEK

sits a fairly large scrap-metal yard that will likely have a few old barges tied to its bulkhead. Stay close to the creek's southern shore to avoid any chance of a run-in between your kayak and one of these rusted hulks.

Past the barges, you'll come to a natural-gas plant on your right, after which the creek begins a sharp turn to the right (south). Follow it as you begin to head almost due south and you'll come to the John Jay Byrne Bridge. Paddle under this bridge, follow the creek as it turns back to the east, and you'll soon be heading straight for the towering Kosciuszko Bridge, which is part of the Brooklyn-Queens Expressway.

Newtown Creek takes on a different feel after the Kosciuszko Bridge as the buildings around it seem to shrink. As a result, the area seems less canyonlike and more open, though all of this changes 0.7 mile later. The creek narrows here and begins the first of six quick, sharp turns that lead deeper into a maze of water, with buildings and bulkheads sitting right on the water's edge. Amazingly, *claustrophobic* is not a word I would use to describe this section of creek. Rather, it's an incredibly interesting place to paddle that seems to be in another world altogether. It may even prove to be the best part of the trip for some. Unfortunately, Newtown Creek comes to an end 1 mile after that first sharp right turn, which leaves only a 3-mile paddle back to your put-in.

✧ **SHUTTLE DIRECTIONS** To get to the put-in at the end of Paige Avenue and Provost Street, take the Long Island Expressway (I-495) to Exit 16 (Greenpoint Avenue). Follow the exit ramp (Borden Avenue) 1 mile before turning left onto Van Dam Street. Take Van Dam Street 0.3 mile until it meets Greenpoint Avenue. Turn right onto Greenpoint Avenue and head west 0.6 mile. Turn right onto Provost Street and follow it to its intersection with Paige Avenue. The waterfront park and boat launch are at the east end of the parking lot, at the intersection's northeastern corner.

 50 NEW YORK UPPER BAY

✧ **OVERVIEW** While it often seems strange to think of New York City in terms of salt water, the entire metropolitan area is, in fact, made up of a series of large and small islands connected to each other via a large network of tidal straits, harbors, bays, and creeks. Taken as a whole, this maritime conglomerate is known as New York Harbor, although it is usually broken up into two main sections: Lower and Upper Bay.

Separated by The Narrows between Staten Island and Brooklyn, these two bays are quite different. The Lower Bay maintains a collection of beaches and other recreational areas, while the Upper Bay is home to the majority of New York Harbor's shipping industry, ferry services, and sightseeing cruises. This greatly increases the amount

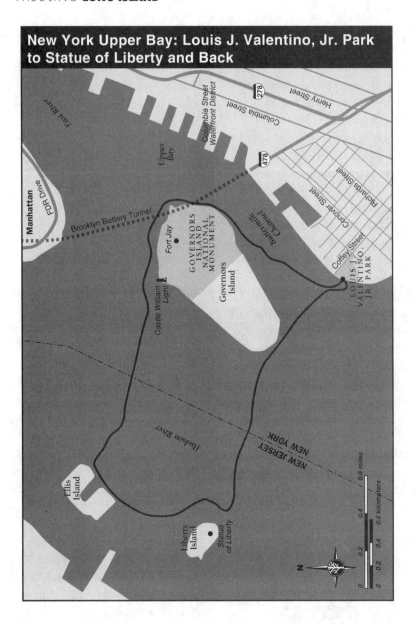

New York Upper Bay: Louis J. Valentino, Jr. Park to Statue of Liberty and Back

of boat traffic—the Upper Bay often seems like a highway during rush hour—but the ships, piers, people, and ports on the bay make it a fascinating place to experience from the water.

Paddle here and you can visit four different islands: Ellis Island, Liberty Island, Governors Island, and Robbins Reef. You can explore the bay mouth's two tributaries, the Hudson River and Gowanus Canal. You can navigate both of its tidal straits, the Kill van Kull and the East River. And you can easily fit the Brooklyn waterfront, Manhattan's southern tip, the South Street Seaport, and

Liberty State Park into a typical day trip's itinerary on the Upper Bay.

Historically, access to the Upper Bay's waters has been limited to private-boat owners, businesses, and those with special permission. But all of that has changed in recent years with the creation of the New York City Water Trail. Five launch sites on the trail provide an easy way to get on the bay: at the northeast corner of Staten Island; in the Brooklyn neighborhood of Red Hook; on the Gowanus Canal, also in Brooklyn; at the northern tip of Governors Island, between southern Manhattan and western Brooklyn; and on Manhattan's Pier 40, on the Hudson in Greenwich Village. Anyone can use these put-ins with the purchase of a $15 annual permit. That all of the Upper Bay is accessible for such a nominal fee only makes it that much more appealing to paddle.

USGS Quadrangles

Jersey City (NJ)

50 **DESCRIPTION** Launch from the pebbly beach at Louis J. Valentino, Jr. Park in Red Hook, and you'll be floating on a small tidal strait called Buttermilk Channel. Legend has it the strait got its name from the dairy farmers who used to row their milk from Brooklyn to Manhattan along its course. Because this water was so rough at times, their milk had been churned enough to turn into buttermilk by the time they got there. Another story holds that strait was once so shallow that cows could be walked directly across from Brooklyn to Governors Island to graze, with the milk being churned within the actual

Louis J. Valentino, Jr. Park to Statue of Liberty and Back

Level	3B
Distance	5.6 miles round-trip
Time	2 hours
Navigable months	Year-round
Hazards	Open water, boat traffic, tidal currents
Portages	None
Rescue access	Difficult
Tidal conditions	Any
Scenery	A+

animals themselves. Regardless of how strait earned its name, you're sure to enjoy paddling along its short length.

Your best bet is to cross Buttermilk Channel and paddle along Governors Island instead of the Brooklyn shore, as the latter is lined with large piers, cranes, barges, and shipping containers. On the other hand, Governors Island boasts tree-lined streets, charming brick buildings, and an incredibly interesting history. It was named *Noten Eylandt* (Dutch for "Island of Nuts") by its first settlers, then renamed Governors Island in 1784 because it was reserved as the exclusive meeting place of the British governors of New

GPS Coordinates

Put-in/take-out
N40° 40.720' W74° 01.101'
Tide station
Gowanus Bay, NY
N40° 39.000' W74° 00.798'

York. It played a big part in the Battle of Long Island, with fortifications that helped hold off the British troops long enough for George Washington's army to escape, and is home to two 19th-century forts, Fort Jay and Castle Williams, both of which served as part of New York's coastal defenses and as military prisons during the Civil War.

Amazingly, both Fort Jay and Castle Williams stand today, near Governors Island's northern tip and its northwestern corner, respectively. Stay close to its shore and you should have no trouble finding either fort. You should also get a great view of Manhattan's South Street Seaport and the Brooklyn Bridge as you look up the East River. Both are only a little more than 1 mile from the tip of Governors Island, close enough for an impromptu paddle

should you have the time. Otherwise, Ellis Island should also be visible almost due west from your position, just 1.5 miles away.

If you want to make the crossing to Ellis Island, you must realize that those 1.5 miles of open water between you and the island can be quite hazardous to paddle at times. Strong tidal currents often flow through the area, just as winds can whip up the surface and create waves of significant height. Combine these conditions with the dozens of passenger ferries, water taxis, cruise ships, tugboats, sailboats, and pleasure craft that zip back and forth across the bay, and it's easy to feel vulnerable out on the water. To combat this feeling, you must paddle strongly and deliberately, making sure that your direction of travel is obvious to all other vessels

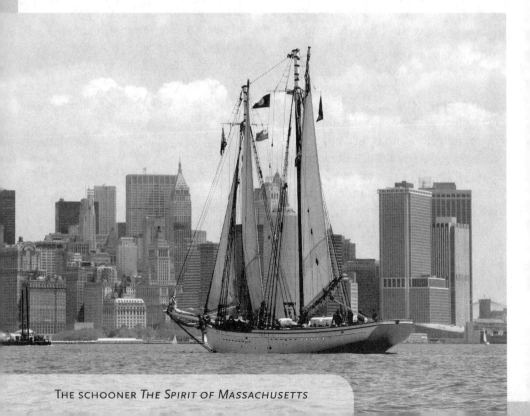

THE SCHOONER *THE SPIRIT OF MASSACHUSETTS*

around you. You should also be patient when performing the crossing, letting any boat larger than you pass before continuing your paddling. The Upper Bay is *not* the place to play chicken or try out the nautical rules of navigation, nor is it the place to tempt your fate with the weather. If the conditions on the water seem to be a bit over your skill or comfort level, don't chance a crossing. But if all factors are in your favor, the chance to see Ellis Island up close is worth the trip.

Most well known as the gateway to the United States for millions of immigrants, Ellis Island is now a 27.5-acre national treasure that is part of the Statue of Liberty National Monument. Truth be told, the island had a less-than-impressive beginning, originating as a 3.5-acre mudflat used for harvesting oysters. Along with a few of its neighboring islands, it was first given the name Oyster Island, although its successive owners renamed it Dyre's, Bucking, and then Anderson's Island. It changed hands again and became Gibbet Island (it was the site of a few hangings). Finally, a man named Samuel Ellis bought the island in 1785 and gave it a name that stuck. He also leased it to New York state, which built a gun battery on it for protection during the War of 1812. A military presence was then maintained on the island for the next 80 years, until it was designated an immigration station in 1892.

As you paddle along Ellis Island, you'll have an amazing view of its main building and its grounds, but be mindful of the security zone set up around its perimeter. You may paddle up to the buoys that mark this perimeter, but you should get no closer than the 150-yard limit they denote. Not to worry—you'll still be close enough to the island to get some great pictures and appreciate its beauty and history.

Once you've had your fill of Ellis Island, head south just 0.5 mile and you'll be floating in the shadow of one of the most recognizable monuments in the world. Standing more than 300 feet high from the base of her pedestal to the top of her crown, the Statue of Liberty is visible from almost every part of New York Harbor, though nothing compares to experiencing her from the seat of a kayak. The detail of her copper skin, the expression on her face, even the writing on her tablet are all easy to see, even while you stay outside of the marked 150-yard security zone.

Frédéric Auguste Bartholdi was the man behind the statue, inspired in 1865 to construct it as a gift from the people of France. Completed 21 years later, it has stood tall on Liberty Island ever since, though not without its problems. Lady Liberty has been closed four times: in 1938, for major renovations; from 1984 to 1986, when the torch and much of the internal structure were replaced; from 2001 to 2009, following the 9/11 attacks (the pedestal reopened in 2004); and from October 2011 to a projected reopening in late 2012, while a secondary staircase and other safety and accessibility features are being added.

After you've had your fill of admiring the Statue of Liberty and snapping photos, it'll be time to turn around and head back to your put-in in Red Hook. Governors Island should be quite easy to spot to the east, but Louis J. Valentino, Jr. Park will probably be out of sight. Head straight for the southern tip of Governors Island, just 1 mile distant. Your view of the Brooklyn shore will improve as you near the island. Once off Governors Island's southern tip, you should be able to spot the large blue-and-yellow Red Hook IKEA store on the Brooklyn waterfront. Head a bit north of the store, and you'll reach your take-out in no time.

◇ **SHUTTLE DIRECTIONS** To get to the put-in at Louis J. Valentino, Jr.

Park in Red Hook, take the Brooklyn-Queens Expressway (I-278) to Exit 26 (Hamilton Avenue). Exit the expressway and take the ramp to Seabring Street. Turn right onto Seabring Street and travel 0.3 mile until you reach Van Brunt Street. Turn left onto Van Brunt Street and drive 0.4 mile before turning right onto Dikeman Street. Go 0.2 mile down Dikeman Street and turn left onto Ferris Street. Take your first right onto Coffey Street and follow it to Louis J. Valentino, Jr. Park, at its end.

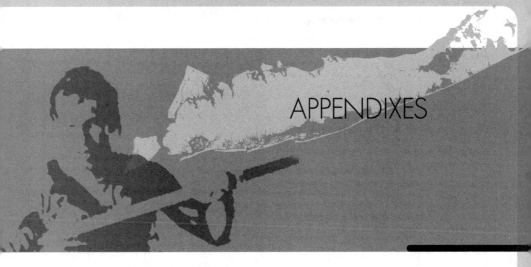

APPENDIX A:
PADDLING OUTFITTERS

SUFFOLK COUNTY

Amagansett Beach and Bicycle Company
624 Montauk Highway
P.O. Box 2483
Amagansett, NY 11930
631-267-6325
amagansettbeachco.com

Rents kayaks and runs guided tours on the South Fork; sells boats, clothing, and paddling gear.

Bob's Canoe Rental, Inc.
631-269-9761
canoerentalslongisland.com

Canoe and kayak rental and livery service on the Nissequogue River.

Captain Kayak–Stein's Marine Center
23 River Road
Sayville, NY 11782
631-750-3587
captainkayak.com

Specializes in sales and rentals of fishing kayaks on the South Shore; offers instruction and tours; sells paddling gear, clothing, and fishing supplies.

Eagle's Neck Paddling Company
62300 Main Road (Route 25)
Southold, NY 11971
631-765-3502
eaglesneck.com

Rents kayaks and runs guided tours on the North Fork; sells boats, clothing, and paddling gear.

Glacier Bay Sports
81-C Fort Salonga Road
Northport, NY 11768
631-262-9116
glacierbaysports.com

Rents kayaks and canoes on the North Shore; sells boats, paddling gear, and clothing.

Nissequogue River Canoe and Kayak Rentals
631-979-8244
canoerentals.com

Rents canoes and kayaks; provides guided tours and instruction on the Nissequogue River.

Peconic Paddler
89 Peconic Ave.
Riverhead, NY 11901
631-727-9895
peconicpaddler.com

Rents canoes and kayaks and provides shuttle services for customers; sells boats and paddling gear.

Setauket Harbor Canoes and Kayaks
30 Shore Road
East Setauket, NY 11733
631-751-2706

Rents kayaks on Setauket and Port Jefferson harbors; sells boats, clothing, and paddling gear.

Shelter Island Kayak Tours
Route 114 at Duvall Street
P.O. Box 360
Shelter Island, NY 11964
631-749-1990
kayaksi.com

Rents kayaks and leads guided tours on Shelter Island.

NASSAU COUNTY

Dinghy Shop
334 S. Bayview Ave.
Amityville, NY 11701
631-264-0005
dinghyshop.com

Rents kayaks and runs guided tours on the South Shore; sells boats, clothing, and paddling gear.

Empire Kayaks
4 Empire Blvd.
Island Park, NY 11558
516-889-8300
empirekayaks.com

Rents kayaks and provides guided tours and instruction in the Island Park——Long Beach area; sells boats, clothing, and paddling gear.

NEW YORK CITY

Long Island City Community Boathouse
718-228-9214
licboathouse.org

Offers free walk-up paddling programs and runs guided tours.

Manhattan Kayak Company
The Boathouse, Pier 66
West 26th Street at 12th Avenue
New York, NY 10001
212-924-1788
manhattankayak.com

Provides kayak rentals, tours, and instruction.

New York City Downtown Boathouse
Box 20214, West Village Station
New York, NY 10014
downtownboathouse.org

Offers free walk-up kayaking programs and guided tours. First-come, first-served.

New York Kayak Company
Pier 40, South Side
West Houston and West streets
New York, NY 10014
800-KAYAK-99
nykayak.com

Offers guided tours; sells canoes, kayaks, paddling gear, and outdoor clothing.

APPENDIX B:
PADDLING CLUBS

Gowanus Dredgers Canoe Club
P.O. Box 22403
Brooklyn, NY 11202
gowanuscanal.org

Inwood Canoe Club
P.O. Box 562
New York, NY 10034
inwoodcanoeclub.org

Kayak Staten Island
kayakstatenisland@gmail.com

Long Island Kayak Club
longislandkayakclub.com

Long Island Paddlers
P.O. Box 115
West Sayville, NY 11796
lipaddlers.org

New York City Downtown Boathouse
Box 20214, West Village Station
New York, NY 10014
downtownboathouse.org

North Atlantic Canoe & Kayak (NACK)
get-the-nack.org

Red Hook Boaters
P.O. Box 24403
Brooklyn, NY 11202-4403
redhookboaters.org

Sebago Canoe Club
Pacrdegat Basin, Foot of Avenue N
Brooklyn, NY 11236
sebagocanoeclub.org

Touring Kayak Club
205 Beach St.
City Island, NY 10464
touringkayakclub.org

Yonkers Paddling and Rowing Club
Alexander Street at Hudson River
Yonkers, NY 10701
yprc.org

APPENDIX C:

ONLINE RESOURCES

American Canoe Association (ACA)
americancanoe.org

Official website of the ACA. Provides information on skills, instruction, stewardship, and membership opportunities as well as lists of publications, outfitters, clubs, and other paddling resources.

Bronx River Alliance
bronxriver.org

Contains a good deal of information about the history and current conditions of the Bronx River. The site also lists valuable information on paddling the Bronx River, such as water conditions and wildlife to look out for.

Campground Owners of New York
nycampgrounds.com

Searchable database of privately owned campgrounds in New York State.

Coast Guard Boating Regulations
uscgboating.org/regulations/
  navigation_rules.aspx

Information on boating regulations and navigation rules.

Metropolitan Transportation
  Authority
mta.info

Provides maps and schedules for bus and subway routes around New York City.

Mobile Geographics
mobilegeographics.com/tides

Online tide tables for most of the globe.

Nassau County Department of Parks,
  Recreation and Museums
1.usa.gov/wQpzKl

List of campgrounds run by Nassau County, with details about locations and reservation policies.

National Oceanic and Atmospheric
  Administration Printable Booklet
  Charts
ocsdata.ncd.noaa.gov/BookletChart

Online database of printable nautical charts, in booklet form.

National Oceanic and Atmospheric
  Administration Tidal Current
  Predictions
tidesandcurrents.noaa.gov

Provides tidal and current predictions for a large number of locations across the United States.

New York City Water Trail
nycgovparks.org/sub_things_to_do/
  facilities/kayak

Gives links to applications for paddling permits and contains an interactive map of the entire New York City Water Trail.

New York State Department of Environmental Conservation
dec.ny.gov

Official website with information on rules and regulations regarding state lands, wildlife, recreation opportunities, maps and facilities, and applications and permits.

New York State Parks
nysparks.com/parks

List of state parks across New York, sorted by available recreational activities or location.

Northeast Paddlers Message Board
npmb.com

Online forum for anyone looking to discuss anything to do with paddling in the northeast United States.

Paddling.net
paddling.net

Online paddling resource containing everything from gear reviews, trip suggestions, dealer listings, and photo galleries to message boards.

Saltwater Tides
saltwatertides.com

Online tide tables for both the East and West coasts of the United States.

Sea Kayaker **Magazine**
seakayakermag.com/PDFs/ float_plan.pdf

Offers a printable template of a paddler's float plan.

Suffolk County Department of Parks, Recreation & Conservation
https://parks.suffolkcountyny.gov/ suffolkcamperweb

List of campgrounds run by Suffolk County, complete with schedules and reservation policies.

United States Geological Survey Water Data
waterdata.usgs.gov/nwis/rt

Online database of water height, flow speed, and temperature for rivers across the United States.

INDEX

ABOUT THE AUTHOR

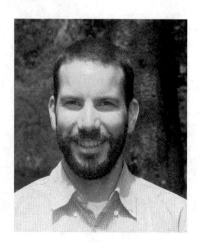

Kevin Stiegelmaier has always been a lover of the outdoors and nature. Growing up on Long Island instilled in him a love of the ocean and led to a degree in marine biology. It also led to the purchase of his first kayak and the beginning of what has been a 14-year passion for paddling. In that time Kevin has canoed and kayaked on every type of water in every state along the East Coast, although he prefers exploring the waters of his home state, New York. Kevin lives on the North Shore of Long Island with his two children, AnnaGrace and William, and teaches high-school biology whenever he isn't paddling. He is also the author of *Canoeing & Kayaking New York* (Menasha Ridge Press).